HOT SPRINGS AND
SPAS
OF CALIFORNIA

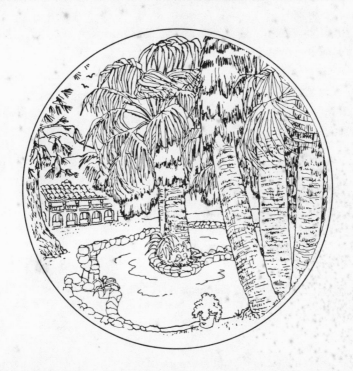

BY PATRICIA COOPER AND LAUREL COOK
DRAWINGS BY FRAN ATTAWAY

101 PRODUCTIONS
SAN FRANCISCO

We gratefully acknowledge the many kindnesses extended to us by the admirable people who staff the spas and resorts we visited. We want to express appreciation to the friends made in each town for their interest and information, and for pointing us down the road to yet another spa. We are grateful to Norma Buferd, who generously assisted early in the project, contributing discriminating observations on Calistoga, Wilbur and Kabuki. Thanks to Willa, Richard and Jenny for their companionship, interest, and continued cheerful assistance. Much appreciation goes to Kim, Erica and Amy who listened, encouraged and supported, each in her own special way, as did Hank, Barbara and Pat.

Special thanks are due Fran Attaway. Her buoyant spirits enlivened our days as much as her drawings enliven the text.—P.C./L.C.

Maps designed and executed by Joan Levi-Kring.

Published by 101 Productions
834 Mission Street, San Francisco, California 94103
Distributed to the book trade in the United States by
Charles Scribner's Sons, New York

Library of Congress Cataloging in Publication Data
Cooper, Patricia.
    Hot springs and spas of California.

    Includes index.
    1. Health resorts, watering-places, etc.—California.
2. Hot springs—California—Guide-books. 3. Mineral
waters—California—Guide-books.   I. Cook, Laurel,
1930- joint author.   II. Title.
RA807.C2C66   613.1'2   78-10665
ISBN 0-89286-145-2

CONTENTS

TAKING THE WATERS 5

NORTHERN CALIFORNIA SPAS 14
  Calistoga Spas, 15
  Calistoga Spa, Calistoga, 19
  Dr. Wilkinson's Hot Springs, Calistoga, 22
  Golden Haven Spa, Calistoga, 26
  Mountain Home Ranch, Calistoga, 29
  Nance's Hot Springs, Calistoga, 32
  Pacheteau's Hot Springs, Calistoga, 36
  Roman Spa, Calistoga, 40
  Wilbur Hot Springs, Wilbur Springs, 42
  Orr Hot Springs, Ukiah, 47
  Campbell Hot Springs, Sierraville, 50
  Family Sauna Shop, San Francisco, 53
  Grand Central Sauna and Hot Tub, San Francisco, 58
  Kabuki Hot Spring, San Francisco, 61
  Albany Sauna, Albany, 66
  American Family Sauna and Tub, Richmond and Oakland, 70
  Berkeley Sauna, Berkeley, 73
  Tassajara Hot Springs, Monterey County, 76
  Esalen Hot Springs, Big Sur, 79

SOUTHERN CALIFORNIA SPAS 82
  The Oaks at Ojai, Ojai, 83
  The Ashram, Calabasas, 88
  Ambassador Tennis and Health Club, Los Angeles, 90
  Glen Ivy Hot Springs, Corona, 92
  Pala Mesa Resort, Fallbrook, 95
  La Costa Spa, Carlsbad, 99
  The Golden Door, Escondido, 104
  Rancho La Puerta, Tecate, Baja California, 110
  Agua Caliente Springs Park, San Diego County, 113
  Warner Hot Springs, San Diego County, 116
  Massacre Canyon Inn, Gilman Hot Springs, 118
  Highland Springs Resort, Beaumont, 122
  Palm Springs Spa Hotel, Palm Springs, 124
  Desert Hot Springs, 128
  Desert Inn, Desert Hot Springs, 133
  Linda Vista Lodge, Desert Hot Springs, 136
  Ponce de Leon Hotel, Desert Hot Springs, 138
  Sam's Family Spa, Desert Hot Springs, 140
  Spa Townhouse, Desert Hot Springs, 142
  The White House, Desert Hot Springs, 144
  Two Bunch Palms, Desert Hot Springs, 147
  Waldorf Health Resort, Desert Hot Springs, 152

INDEX 154

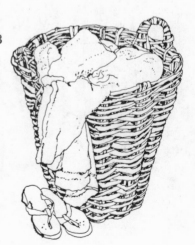

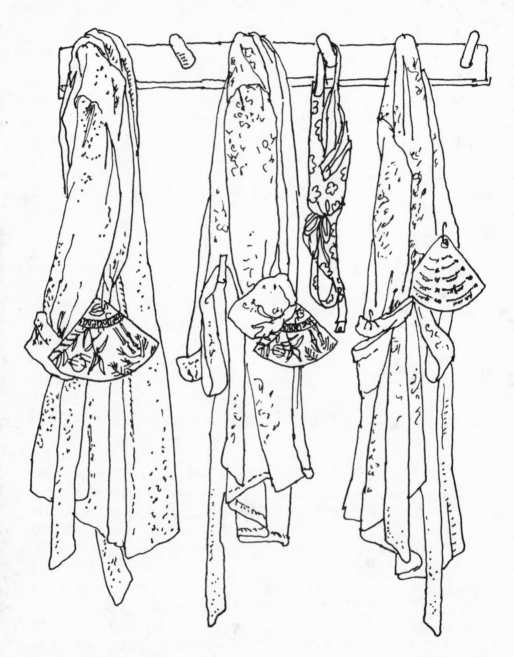

Robes hang at the Golden Door spa.

TAKING THE WATERS

This book is to introduce and guide you to taking the waters in California. When the project was conceived four years ago, our intention was to tell readers about country sources of natural thermal springs where they could discover, as we had, the joys of relaxing neck-deep in hot mineral waters. Since that time, there has been a renewed awareness in the United States that hot water is pleasurable as well as therapeutic for body and mind. With that recognition has come a proliferation of spas and health resorts, encouraging us to broaden our perspective to include both urban and country facilities.

We have retained our original focus on water soaking as the prime experience, and the newcomer to the waters as our primary audience. But we know that those who have savored the deep relaxation and simple joy of soaking in hot water or luxuriated in the heat of sauna and steam will also find this book a valuable resource for future explorations into spas and hot springs.

The diversity of places to take the waters in California is truly astounding. Our selection is not comprehensive, but is based on our desire to present a wide variety of spa experiences. What we looked for was *water*—whether city water heated and piped into hot tubs, or mineral water welling up from deep in the earth to erupt at the surface as steamy geysers and boiling hot springs.

In country locations, we confined our reviews to those places that offer accommodations, either on the premises or immediately adjacent. Whether in the city or country, we included only those spas open for public use. Our final concern was that readers be given a range of prices—from inexpensive overnight camping fees of the state park mineral pools to elaborate week-long programs in California's most luxurious spa resorts.

In some spas, the only attraction is hot water in pools and tubs. In others, a hot soak is but one of numerous health and relaxation activities offered from a list that includes sauna, steam, massage and mud bath. In the spas which stress fitness along with health and relaxation, the list lengthens to include tennis, golf, horseback riding, structured exercise programs and yoga.

Whether the facility provides only tub soaks under the redwoods or a full resort atmosphere of vacation activity, all from the most rustic to the most splendid, are in business to provide you with an opportunity to refresh and renew body, mind and spirit.

Newcomers to the waters often have questions about spa protocol. How much privacy can I expect to have? Will I be nude in front of others? Will I find people my age? Will they expect me to know the routines?

Believe it or not, after one or two visits to spas, these questions simply evaporate. The spa experience is a natural one, not exotic as many newcomers seem to think. Most of the people you will encounter are there to make their bodies feel good—for an hour out of their busy days or for a week out of their lives. You will soon find that you are free to move through the spa experience as you wish. In most places, you are given a wrap of some kind, a cotton robe, a kimono, or a large sheet or towel for moving from one activity to another. When you are soaking in a tub or taking a sauna, you can wear a bathing suit if it makes you feel more comfortable. In the more elaborate spas where an attendant leads you around, you will be slipping in and out of wraps and sheets for your tub and massage, and we can only tell the body-shy that nudity is simply not a problem. The point is for *you* and your body to feel good.

The best clue to the routines of a given spa will be found in the text for that spa. Generally, we would suggest that you take time to read the literature at the desk or posted in the tub and sauna rooms, and then, ask questions. Attendants and spa staff are used to questions. It is their daily job to meet the public and to be helpful in seeing them through the spa. They may suggest to you, for example, how long it is advisable to remain in the sauna, or when to pour water over the rocks in small dipper quantities. But in the last analysis, you must listen to your own body. We each have different tolerances for heat and what is deliciously warm to one may be uncomfortably hot to another.

Another question often asked is about gratuities. The tipping policies and protocol vary enormously from spa to spa; inquire at the desk as you register.

Some hot spring resorts have unusual routines. Tassajara, for example, is primarily a Buddhist monastery and school. You are not required to follow the routine of the monks and students, but you are expected to respect the spirit of a monastic community. At Calistoga, all the spas offer similar routines in the bathhouse, and the staff may matter-of-factly usher you from hot mineral tub to mud bath if you have signed up for the works. If you prefer to rest awhile, or to stop for a drink of fruit juice, just say so. The routine should never intrude on your sense of leisure and well-being.

The overgrown ruins of Fetters Hot Springs near Calistoga.

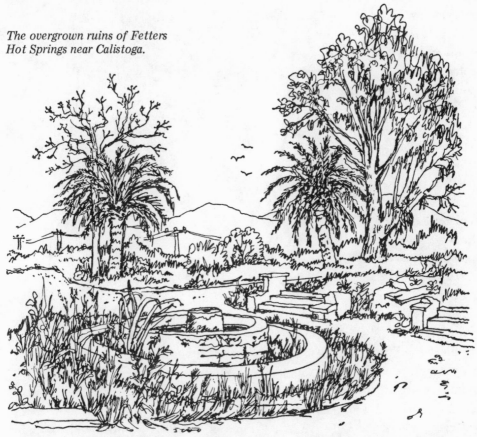

Once you have visited a couple of spas, you will probably join the aficionados who have their bags packed and ready for the one-hour vacation of a city spa or the more extended visit to a country hot spring. One of the nicest things about the spa sport is that your paraphernalia can be as simple or as elaborate as you choose. While most spas furnish the equipment and provide towels and sheets, we have developed over time what we refer to as "The Basic Bag."

7

"Let all my children drink of its waters . . ."
—Chief Morongo, Morongo Springs.

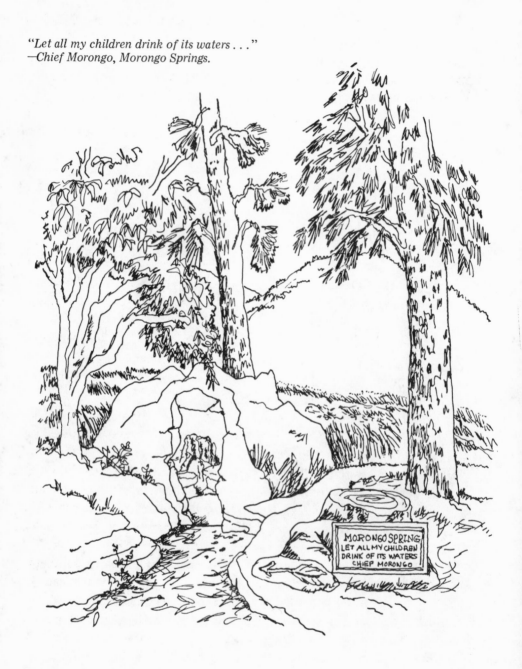

Into the bag go all those things that over a lifetime have come to mean real comfort and relaxation (even pampering) to you. Through the years, we have seen veteran spa-goers pull out exotic lotions, moldy sun visors, sketch pads, blow-up toys, mineral-ion fortified drinks from plastic flight bags, cardboard boxes, Gucci pouches, and backpacks . . . part of their Basic Bag.

Dress is usually informal at all spas, unless you go in for night life, so put clothes on your back or in a suitcase and reserve your Basic Bag for items associated with bathing and relaxation. Some items:

• A thin nylon bathing suit, for spas that require clothing in the pools, will keep weight to a minimum and dry quickly.

• A shower cap or bathing cap for appropriate times.

• A lightweight kimono that folds flat into a small space—made of cotton, soft as skin, and most useful in spa transitions where bare is not beautiful or even allowed.

• A thin, nylon parka that rolls into a small space. Rarely used, it serves well when stepping out of a natural hot spring into the cool night air of country or desert.

• Unbreakable bottles and tubes of moisturizers, shampoo, rinse and hair conditioners, cologne, make-up, comb and brush, and a manicure set.

• Sandals or zoris, with soles that will hold up while walking short distances over stones.

And last, but not least, carry a thermometer in an unbreakable case for measuring water temperature. While this suggestion may sound farfetched to the novice, experienced soakers find they want to know by their own measure the temperature of water or sauna. Some bathers feel best in water of 105 degrees; others know they do not tolerate high temperatures well and prefer to stay around 100 degrees. Unless there is a thermometer attached to the pool or sauna, it's hard to know, even with the elbow test, how to time your stay. A favorite question on the edge of the pool is, "How hot is it?" Five people invariably give five different answers—with the management chiming in for a sixth.

After a little experience, you will know exactly the temperature and time suited to your body, to your own states of stress, tension and blood pressure, to your own sense of well-being.

Hot springs have relaxed and delighted man throughout recorded history and references to hot mineral springs are found throughout the history of California. The records of settlers using hot springs as health retreats in the state begins in the late 19th century. Homesteaders from Europe, where for centuries people had put great faith in the medicinal and therapeutic value of thermal springs, began to duplicate the spas that were familiar to them, using the natural abundance of hot spring waters in California. Often they shared the use of the springs with American Indians who used the hot mineral waters that came from the ground and revered their healing powers. Spanish settlers proclaimed the springs *agua caliente,* "hot water," a name still on streets and spas throughout California.

Most of the city spas were started by the Finnish who sought to duplicate the community sauna that was part of their childhood in the old country or in Finnish communities in the United States. American entrepreneurs attracted to the health spa concept generally followed the lead offered by the Finnish for whom the communal sauna was a daily aspect of family life. It is said that the Finns put together their sauna before they built their main house. Today, such spas as Albany Sauna, Berkeley Sauna, American Family Sauna and Family Sauna carry on the Finnish tradition in the San Francisco Bay Area.

Kabuki Hot Springs in Japan Center in the heart of San Francisco, on the other hand, duplicates traditional Japanese practices, including their famed shiatsu, or deep thumb-pressure massage. In Japan, as in Finland, the tradition of family communal bathing has a long history. It is worth repeating the adage "Americans bathe to get clean; Japanese get clean to bathe" for it is a practice you will be expected to honor at Kabuki, as well as at other spas where communal bathing occurs. Kabuki separates its men's and women's quarters, and unlike the Finnish sauna, a Japanese attendant guides you every step of the way, scrubbing your back, leading you from tub to sauna to massage.

In the California countryside a number of the older spas were designed at the turn of the century to resemble the famous resorts of Central Europe— Baden-Baden and Karlsbad. Many of the country spas are still European-owned or managed and cater to a European clientele. You will find this continental influence in Calistoga, in the contoured tubs of Gilman Hot Springs and in the health regimes of Desert Hot Springs.

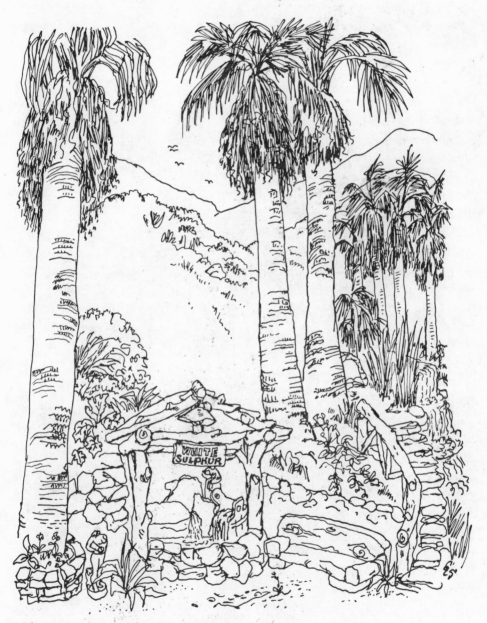

Sulphur springs grotto, Soboba Hot Springs.

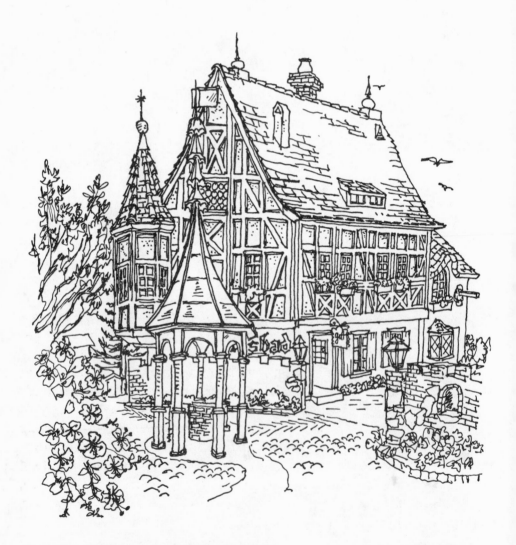

The well at Alt Karlsbad Hanse House, Carlsbad,
dug in 1882. Analysis proved the water to be like
the Ninth Spa at Karlsbad, Bohemia.

Throughout Southern California, historical markers repeatedly remind you that the Indians first discovered the healing quality of water in this country, and later taught the Spanish settlers the curative use of *agua caliente*. If you look closely, you will see clear evidence of the evolution from Indian to Spanish to European to modern use of hot spring sites.

Five minutes north of Gilman Hot Springs is historic Soboba Hot Springs, no longer open to the public and now privately run as a transcendental meditation center. Nevertheless the owners graciously invited us for a look around. The old mineral water pool stands quietly in its ruins, eroded by multiple underground springs that have made their impression on the landscape. California Indian and early Spanish influences are seen in the simple adobe buildings around the spring, and in the blood-red bougainvillea draping the old bathhouse. If you walk uphill through brambles and thickets, you will find an old grotto housing an image of the Virgin Mary, placed there to bless the waters—an echo of hope and homage to the waters.

Another vestige of California's historic spas is the town of Carlsbad, so named because an analysis from the first well dug here in 1882 revealed that the mineral waters approximated those of the "Ninth Spa of Karlsbad" in Bohemia. Germans, Bohemians and English settled Carlsbad, rather than the Spanish who influenced so much of our state. The waters are no longer a major attraction, but this site of the well is a testimonial to the founding fathers of Carlsbad. In the basement of the Alt Karlsbad's Hanse House a handsome German building, the original mineral well is still on view, surrounded by the replica of a gazebo from the Ninth Spa of Karlsbad.

The history of other hot springs in California is interwoven throughout this book in individual descriptions of the spas. As you go from spa to spa you will discover for yourself colorful bits of California history.

Our first wish, however, is that you *experience* all the varieties of water and massage: Finnish wet and dry saunas, soothing Swedish massage, invigorating shiatsu and gentle, modern, American Esalen massage. Relax deeply in an individual, body-contoured European tub, soak with your friends in a communal Japanese tub. Sink into a quiet, natural pool under the open sky . . . unwind, enjoy.

Patricia Cooper
Laurel Cook
Berkeley, 1978

NORTHERN CALIFORNIA

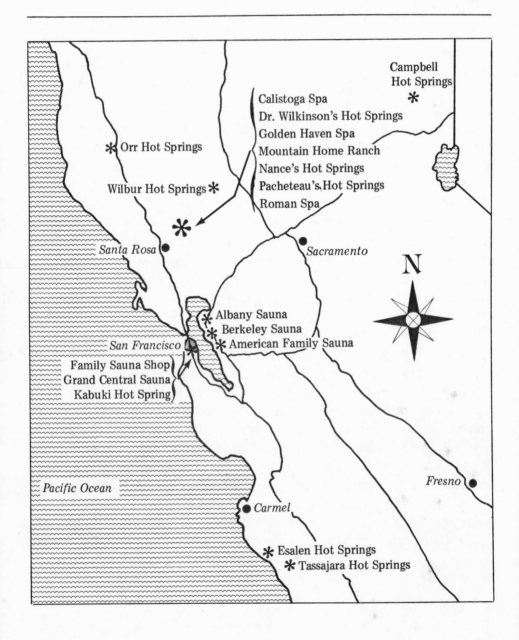

Campbell Hot Springs
*

Calistoga Spa
Dr. Wilkinson's Hot Springs
Golden Haven Spa
Mountain Home Ranch
Nance's Hot Springs
Pacheteau's Hot Springs
Roman Spa

* Orr Hot Springs

Wilbur Hot Springs *

*

Santa Rosa ●

● Sacramento

N

* Albany Sauna
* Berkeley Sauna
San Francisco
* American Family Sauna

Family Sauna Shop
Grand Central Sauna
Kabuki Hot Spring

Pacific Ocean

Fresno ●

● Carmel

* Esalen Hot Springs
* Tassajara Hot Springs

CALISTOGA SPAS
Napa Valley

The hot springs and health spas of the Calistoga area deserve a prelude. Calistoga, located in Napa County, is the repository of natural delights worth pages of description.

Situated in the heart of California wine country, neighbor to the finest vineyards and wineries, Calistoga sits atop what appears to be an unlimited supply of hot mineral water welling from mysterious sources deep in the earth to surface displays of great variety—shooting geysers, hissing steam vents, boiling hot ponds and deep, tepid mineral pools.

Were this not blessing enough, the air is clear. Napa Valley light playing off the green hills and valley floor has a quality all its own. Everywhere the brown, knarred vines of Chardonnay, Pinot Noir and Cabernet Sauvignon grapes grow in manicured lines. Rolling hills are dotted with groves of giant oak, tangles of madrone and flowering shrubs, groups of cows and horses.

The area was settled beginning in the 1830s, and many of the original buildings erected in the 19th century are still in use or have been restored as museums. The window into the pioneer heritage of California seems always open in the Napa Valley, preserved not only in the architecture and the vineyards, but in the gentle vigorous life style.

At the turn of the century, some 70 years after early pioneers began to edge the Pomos and Mayacamas Indians out of the valley, the countryside in a 50-mile radius of Calistoga was graced with some 30 separate vigorously growing resorts. Each was centered around mineral springs and complete with wooden hotel, verandas, cabins, stately grounds and elaborate bathhouses. In the case of Calistoga Spa, there was a thriving horse race track. People came to the resorts from all over California, but especially from San Francisco via ferry, horse-drawn coach or steam train, and on the last legs of the journey by carriage and horseback.

By 1930, most of these resorts and spas had succumbed to fire, financial reversals and the change in fashion from country to urban entertainment. Calistoga Hot Springs and the spa motels are built on the remains of the era, and are currently responding to the renaissance in spa resorts by remodeling existing facilities and planning new spas.

The original spas, like today's motel spas, were devoted to health and relaxation. The earliest guides to mineral springs in Calistoga were published in 1890 and report "These springs have obtained considerable reputation for their healing properties. It is claimed that an agreeable softness of the skin is obtained by external use of the waters. The water is also used for rheumatism, scrofula, constitutional taints, and internal complaints." Each of these old descriptions includes a careful analysis of the mineral content of the water, as well as a description of the temperature range of springs issuing from the earth. The faintly therapeutic and medicinal air of the spas of yesteryear still mingles with the modest and hedonistic claims made by modern Calistoga spas.

Like their counterpart in the South, The Desert Hot Springs, Calistoga baths originate in natural hot mineral springs, and most spas have wells and extensive holding tanks on their premises. One of the characteristics of a Calistoga morning is the sight of white vapors and hot jets of steam rising into the cool air from the mineral-encrusted vents and pipes behind the spas which line the main street.

Another characteristic of Calistoga Spas is the Calistoga mud bath, a mixture of volcanic ash and mineral water—thick, black, odoriferous and bubbling—into which you ease your wary body for bone-penetrating warmth and relaxation.

The resort spas of Calistoga are built in conventional motel style. There is no pretention to glamour or luxury; rather the facilities are functional and devoted in atmosphere and design to the hot waters they provide. Each motel has a series of hot tubs, baths and steam rooms which are housed in a complex adjacent to the individual rooms or cottages where guests live. The bathhouses, usually situated right over the hot springs or near the voluminous holding tanks for mineral waters, are redolent of sulphur and other exotic mineral smells. In the older bathhouses, the mineral-encrusted pipes are exposed around the edges of wooded floors, spitting steam and coughing smoke. One assumes they are a direct pipeline to hell.

Your motel bathroom is also piped from these underground springs in Calistoga. You can drink Calistoga water right from your kitchen faucet and

The bridge to the natural hot pool.
The Geysers, Geyserville.

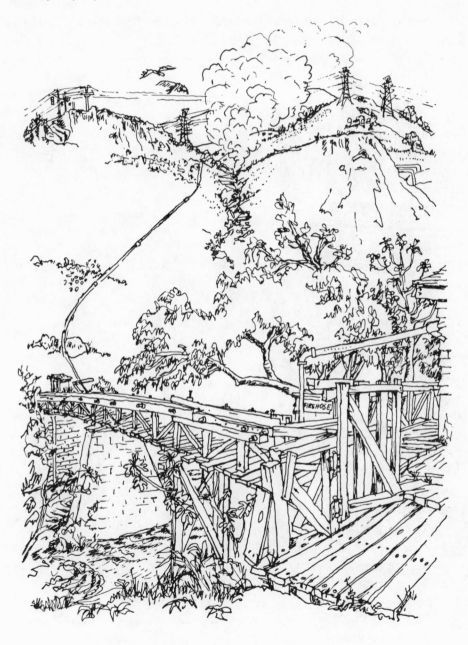

save the price of 30 cents a glass at the local bar. Draw a really hot tub the minute you hit your room after a deadening week in the city, and sink immediately into the steamy, soothing atmosphere of this amazing little California town.

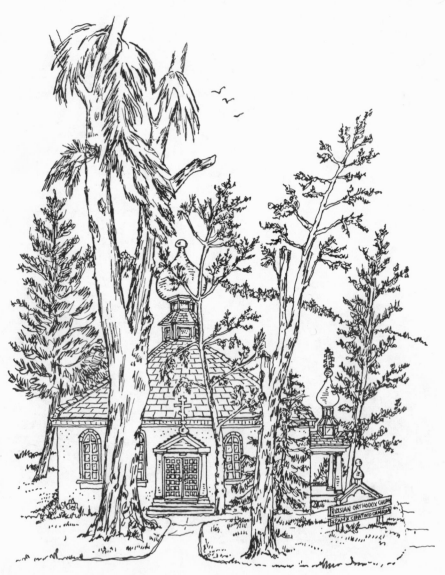

Russian Orthodox Church with golden domes, Calistoga.

CALISTOGA SPA
Calistoga

The special charm of Calistoga Spa lies in the friendliness and attentiveness of its manager and staff. The Barretts, who manage the spa, have been in the business for years and they are the perfect guides to an introduction to hot water bathing. They, or one of the staff, will take you on a tour of the premises, showing you the facilities and explaining all procedures.

As Calistoga Spa is fairly typical of all the spas in town, a quick run through their accommodations and programs will give you a thumbnail tour of the town. Calistoga excels in the use of hot mineral waters and volcanic-ash mud baths. You may take the waters in tubs, steam rooms, saunas, outdoor pools, internally, and in all temperatures from boiling hot to ice cold. Mud baths are taken only one way, hot and submerged in a large concrete tub; more about mud is scattered among the other spa descriptions. This spa has a team of skilled massage therapists, as do most of the spas in town. Hot blanket wraps and cooling showers complete the treatment of a typical program in Calistoga.

The atmosphere of Calistoga Spa is lively. This is a popular spa, booked up for lodgings six months in advance, with many clients returning again and

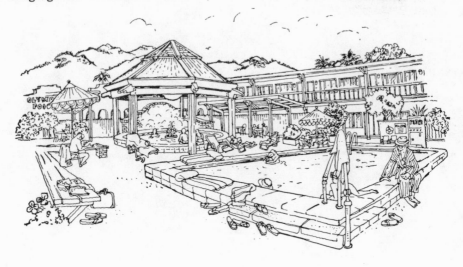

again. Said one acquaintance turning slowly and rhythmically from side to side in the hydrojets, "I've come here every Saturday for the last 10 years. I've got a tough job, and I haven't been sick a day in 40 years; I do believe it's due to these waters. In just two years I've seen these waters become so popular that the place is blooming with new buildings. Half of the people here are young people; I say it's like the old days . . . before the wars."

Around the two big outdoor hot pools, people move to and fro about their spa business or seem absorbed in books and conversation, sun visors and sun glasses firmly in place. There are always family groups at Calistoga Spa, and parties of students up from area colleges. A certain pleasant camaraderie prevails.

A soak in these large outdoor tubs at Calistoga Spa makes the perfect ending to a day in the wine country. The spa is open until nine o'clock, but for a small fee you can soak under the stars, tucked in warm water up to your chin.

Inside the bathhouse, men and women have separate quarters, and this is as good a place as any to face up to your first mud bath. Begin by standing over the tub. Contemplate the oozing, bubbling surface—ancient, wet, volcanic ash. Allow your imagination certain rein regarding this huge mud pie—think of it as mud between the toes—that familiar, bracing thought should get you ankle deep and sitting way back on the tub edge.

At this point in your initiation, the attendant will say "Just tilt in now,"

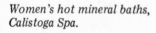
Women's hot mineral baths, Calistoga Spa.

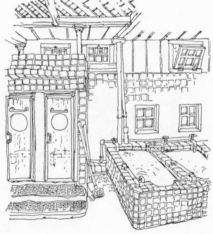

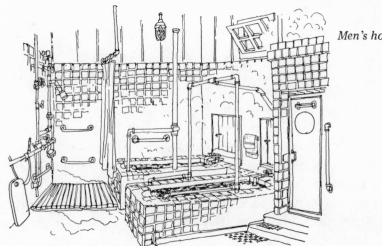

*Men's hot mineral baths,
Calistoga Spa.*

and to your amazement, your body will begin to disappear beneath your eyes, inch-after-inch devoured by the earth. Truly, as they claim, the heat is most penetrating and relaxing. You remain an allotted 15 minutes and emerge, caked and blackened, slop over to the showers, and end the ordeal with a sluice of tepid mineral water.

Hot mineral whirlpool baths and steam cabinets follow the mud bath. When you are out of the last water treatment, your attendant will wrap you in warm flannel blankets in a private room where you will remain until called for your massage.

Accommodations at Calistoga Spa include rooms and cottages surrounding the large spa building. Some of the cottages are equipped with kitchens, utensils and dishes; all the rooms have television and private baths. Convenient to the shops, restaurants, post office of main street, this is the spa we would recommend for stays which last longer than a weekend in Calistoga.

CALISTOGA SPA, 1006 Washington Street, Calistoga, California 94515. Telephone: (707) 942-6269. Accommodations: rooms and cottages; private baths; single, double, queen-size beds; some fully equipped kitchens. Rates: singles from $18, doubles from $21. No meal service. Reservations recommended. Children and pets welcome. Cards: BA, MC. Open all year.
Spa facilities: hot outdoor pools, Jacuzzi, $3 per day, free to overnight guests; mineral bath, steam room, blanket wrap, $8, with mud bath, $10; massage, $15. Bathing suits required for all communal baths; suits optional in separate men's and women's quarters.

DR. WILKINSON'S HOT SPRINGS
Calistoga

The large, imposing neon sign announcing Dr. Wilkinson's Hot Springs beckons at the end of Lincoln Avenue, Calistoga's main street. The most prominent of the street's neons, the sign looks most inviting on a foggy, cold winter night after a tiring week's work in San Francisco.

The building presents a neat, concrete block and sparkling glass facade, a preface to the spare, modern interior. The spa contains the newest, freshest equipment and accommodations in Calistoga. Dr. Wilkinson has been on this corner for several decades, and he is constantly improving and updating his facility.

Dr. Wilkinson is a chiropractor, and his emphasis on health and well-being together with his professional attitude, gives this place more of a therapeutic air than others in Calistoga. The atmosphere is one of a small, friendly, attentive clinic or hospital—at least from the outside and in the foyer. Once inside the bathhouse and inner courtyards, this aura is somewhat dispelled by the warm redwood decor, spacious mirrored dressing rooms and wonderful greenhouse-enclosed hot pool.

Dr. Wilkinson's, over the years, has enjoyed a growing reputation for efficient service and a serious concern with health. The program here involves hot water baths only, or a combination of massage, chiropractic adjustment and physical therapy (by a registered physical therapist).

We were greeted at the desk on our latest visit by Dr. Wilkinson's son, Mark, who told us that, indeed, the business is family run. "We've been helping out since we were children," he commented, gesturing to a framed children's drawing showing all the kids at Dad's spa, painted by the Wilkinson children some years back. Mark is enthusiastic about the spa business, eager to answer questions, so we asked our favorite: "What is a mud bath?" He's heard the question and answered it so many times that he's had mud bath cards printed to hand customers.

"The Mud Bath consists of a white volcanic ash powder, found in the Calistoga area, mixed in with the naturally heated mineral water which is so abundant here. This mixture produces a thick, warm, heavy mud in which

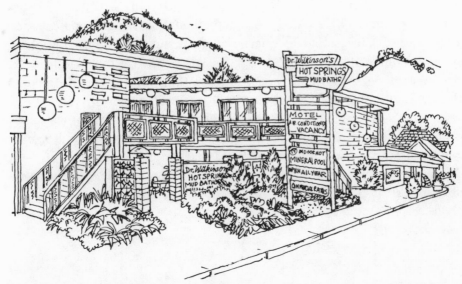

the bather is completely immersed. Generally, you stay in for 10 to 15 minutes, then into the mineral baths. You take a mud bath because it is relaxing, drawing out toxins in the system, cleansing the skin. You perspire heavily in the hot mud resulting in further cleansing. Also the mud is clinging, and for people with muscular aches the heat of the mud seems particularly penetrating, soothing and relaxing."

The bathhouses for men and women are separate. We went through the simple bath routine here, and were particularly impressed with the attentive staff who assisted us out of the steam rooms and into warm blanket wraps for an hour's nap. Massage, expertly performed, followed. Then we moved outside to the communal pool.

The big hot-water pool is located just outside the bathhouse in a large glass-enclosed room. The whole place feels like the interior of a greenhouse —steamy, humid and completely welcoming. The roof is lined with redwood beams, the floor and walls contain planters filled with fruit trees, bamboo, flowering bushes, azalea and magnolia—a small paradise. Slide into the pool, lie back against a Jacuzzi jet and gaze out the open doors to the dreamy blue-green of the surrounding mountains.

Rooms here have kitchens, color cable television, air conditioning, and ready access to the courtyards and parking. There is also a small conference room at this spa. They welcome seminars and group meetings.

DR. WILKINSON'S HOT SPRINGS, 1507 Lincoln Avenue, Calistoga 94515. Telephone: (707) 942-4102. Accommodations: rooms and cottages; private baths; single, double, queen-size beds; no telephones; television; some fully equipped kitchens. Rates: $22 single to $34 for four; kitchens, $4 extra; weekly rates. No meal service. Reservations recommended. Children welcome. Cards: BA, MC. Conference facilities for 25. Open all year.

Spa facilities: Hot mineral pool, Jacuzzi, $1 per day for overnight guests, $4 per day for non-guests; mud bath, mineral bath, steam room and blanket wrap, $10; massage and mineral bath, $16. Chiropractic adjustment, $12. Bathing suits required in all communal pools; suits optional in separate men's and women's baths.

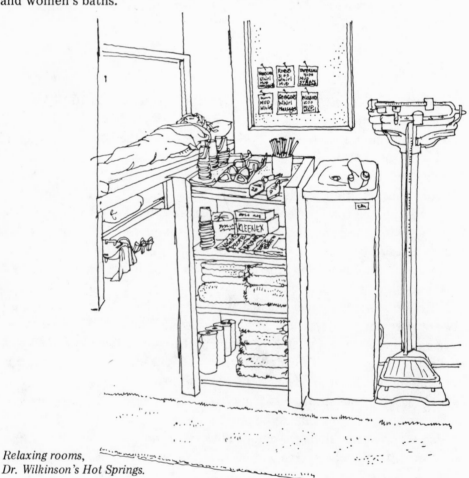

Relaxing rooms,
Dr. Wilkinson's Hot Springs.

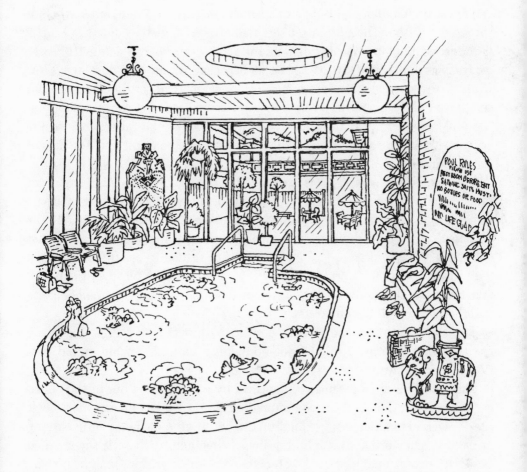

Hot mineral water pool,
Dr. Wilkinson's Hot Springs.

GOLDEN HAVEN SPA
Calistoga

A ritual of note among lovers of the California country scene is the annual trip to the Napa County Fair in Calistoga during the first week in July. We stayed at the Golden Haven Spa one Fourth of July weekend, and a haven it turned out to be. The uproar on the main drag of Calistoga over the Fourth is exceeded only by the pandemonium at the fairgrounds some 10 blocks away. Beer and wine flow; the haze of barbecue smoke and dust hangs low over the town; campers, vans, motorcycles and cars cruise around. Our semi-sane solution was to bring our bicycles and walking shoes, hole up at the Golden Haven, and walk or cycle from town to the fairgrounds to the spas, returning for a quiet breather to the silence, seclusion and hot tubs of the Haven.

The Golden Haven Spa is located 10 blocks off the main street of Calistoga on a tree-lined, small-town thoroughfare. The low, green frame buildings of the spa blend into the quiet, residential neighborhood. At the entrance, as a small drive widens into a parking lot, you feel you've just entered a friend's driveway. The grounds are intimate, beautifully planted with roses, honeysuckle and jasmine. Flowering trees lean out over the pools, and the small bungalows immediately in sight have private patios complete with barbecue grills for cookouts.

The air of intimacy and charm continues into the pool area. Big shade trees border a large, roofed pool containing natural, unchlorinated, unfiltered mineral water.

This same water, constantly replenished by a flow in and out of the pools, is found also in the outdoor, communal redwood tub. The management took the time to explain carefully some of the advantages of therapeutic bathing in natural, unchlorinated sulphur springs. Prime among these is the sensible observation that unchlorinated water does not dry the skin, making it flake and peel. Chlorine irritates the delicate membranes of the eyes and the nasal membranes; natural spring water does not. In addition, these mineral waters, though sulfurous, have a nice fresh smell.

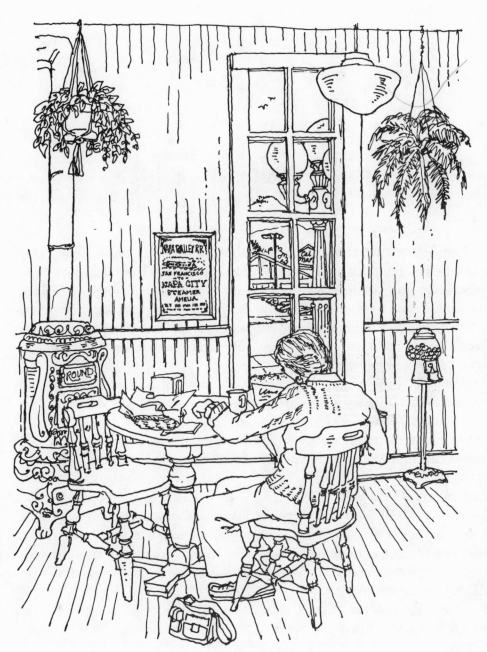

Cafe in the restored railroad station, Calistoga.

Public mineral water swimming pool, Calistoga.

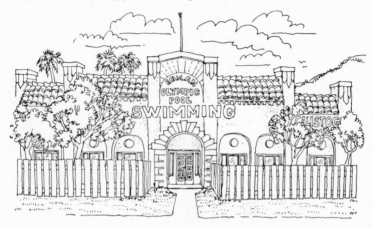

Reflexology foot massage is a featured therapy at the Golden Haven. Tiny pressure points on the foot are worked over in detail by the skilled hands of Miss Quinn, the resident massage therapist. She explains every detail of the procedure, so do ask questions. Essentially Miss Quinn says a good massage should leave you feeling warmer, more elongated, lighter and more supple. You should have a sensation of increased warmth in the deep muscles due to an increase in blood circulation.

The full body massage combines techniques of Swedish massage and pressure-point massage. The most luxurious treatment is a one-hour foot massage and a half-hour of back, neck and shoulder massage.

Rooms surround the courtyard and hot pools. They are average, clean and neat motel rooms; most have kitchens and all have television.

GOLDEN HAVEN SPA, 1713 Lake Street, Calistoga, California 94515. Telephone: (707) 942-5296. Accommodations: rooms and cottages; private baths; single, double, queen-size beds; no telephones; television; many fully equipped kitchens. Rates: $22 single to $36 for four. No meal service. Reservations recommended. Children welcome. Some pets allowed. Cards: AE, BA, MC. Open all year.
Spa facilities: outdoor mineral pool, hot tubs, Jacuzzi, $5 per day, free to overnight guests; $15 foot massage, $12.50 back massage. Bathing suits required.

MOUNTAIN HOME RANCH
Calistoga

If you wish to combine a vacation with children and a trip to the Calistoga spas, consider staying at Mountain Home Ranch. While not a hot-water spa, this is the perfect place to satisfy kids out for country fun, as well as adults who want to soak, golf, hike or just sit around in a beautiful wooded environment. A short six-mile drive takes you into the spas at Calistoga. The staff at Mountain Home Ranch were themselves children on this ranch, following two generations of family before them, and they know exactly what appeals to youngsters around this neck of the woods. The place is homey, the food is delicious, and as the manager says, "The main idea is to shed your cares and have fun."

To reach Mountain Home Ranch, from Calistoga take Highway 128 north and turn left on the Petrified Forest Road. The road plunges you instantly into the peace and quiet of rural life. Winding up the mountain past manicured vineyards and small fenced pastures, stop under a tall eucalyptus tree or in a grove of oaks, bring out the wine and cheese, spread a blanket and picnic. Slow down. The countryside alone is worth the trip.

Continue on up the road and turn right at the sign for Mountain Home Ranch, drive two miles to the site of the Ranch, and feast your eyes on a view of the Napa valley and the mountains beyond. The peak of Mt. St. Helena is visible in the clear air.

Settling into the hospitality of Mountain Home Ranch for us means taking leisurely walks and sunbathing. But you can be as active as you care to with swimming, fishing, horseback riding and a golf course 10 minutes away. If you like to hike, begin with a slow amble along the creek shaded by willows and redwoods, before striking off into the trails which crisscross the surrounding wooded mountains.

Mountain Home Ranch shares a rich pioneer heritage with the rest of the Calistoga area. Today the resort is managed by the third generation of the Orth family who were original homesteaders on this land in the late 19th century. Emma and Ludwig Orth were among the many European pioneers

...o traveled westward seeking land of their own. They settled on 80 acres which is now the ranch, later buying adjacent land to increase their spread. At first the family lived in a one-room log cabin near the small stream which meanders through the ranch. Ludwig went to work 60 miles away in Richmond, and every Friday night he came home to Calistoga by steam train, walking the six uphill miles to the ranch carrying the week's supply of staples in a backpack.

At that time the family table was not spread with the good fried chicken and table wines of today, but with squirrel and rabbit from the woods.

By 1914 when the Orths were able to invest in a horse and buggy, friends had begun to visit the ranch regularly, especially in the summer, from Oakland, Richmond and San Francisco. They slept in tents, swam in the creek, hiked the hills and ate together at one long table on the screened porch of what is now the main ranch building.

By the 1940s, Emma Orth, the Orths' only daughter, had taken over the 400-acre ranch and the management of the resort. Today children of Emma manage Mountain Home Ranch and raise the fourth generation to remain on the land.

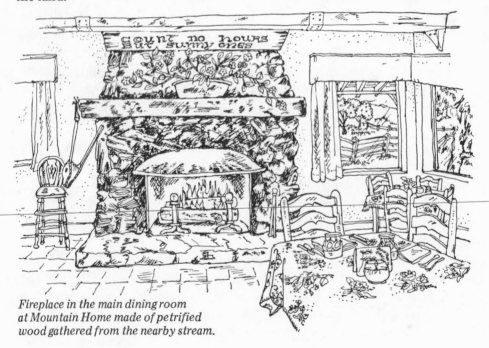

Fireplace in the main dining room at Mountain Home made of petrified wood gathered from the nearby stream.

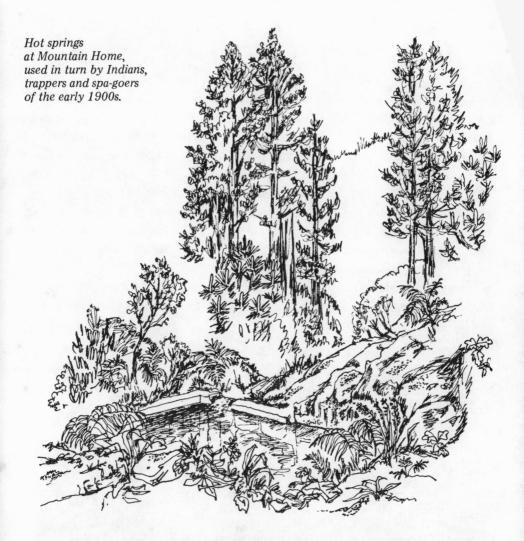

Hot springs
at Mountain Home,
used in turn by Indians,
trappers and spa-goers
of the early 1900s.

MOUNTAIN HOME RANCH, 3400 Mountain Home Ranch Road, Calistoga, California 94515. Telephone: (707) 942-6616. Accommodations: rooms in main lodge, rustic summer cabins; some private baths, some shared; single, double beds; television. Rates: $18 to $27 single, $30 to $42 double, breakfast and dinner included; $16 to $20, no meals; special children's rates. Reservations recommended. Children and pets welcome. Cards: BA, MC. Open all year.
Facilities: swimming, fishing, hiking, horseback riding; no spa facilities.

NANCE'S HOT SPRINGS
Calistoga

At first appearance Nance's is an average-size motel, typical in appearance and room plan to any 1930s roadside oasis. The pale, cream stucco exterior and red-tiled roof, of course, signal its California location. But just inside— Aha! Shazam! A California mineral-bath heaven.

The two outer wings of motel rooms and offices shelter the bathhouse and inner courtyard, the latter centered with a steaming pool and lined with walkways through banana and palm trees. The bathhouse continues back over a half-block area, with men's quarters on one side and women's on the other, a typical arrangement in Calistoga spas.

Where one would expect to find a coffee shop and convention rooms in a conventional motel, at Nance's a hydrojet, natural-spring-water, communal

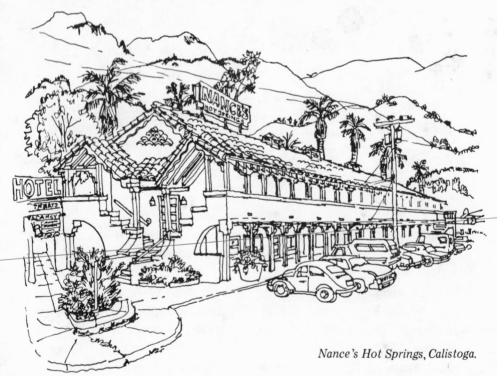

Nance's Hot Springs, Calistoga.

hot tub bubbles and steams vigorously. Enclosed in a glass house, with sliding doors open on one side to the inner courtyard, the tub is irresistible. We entered the glass house one recent Saturday afternoon to find people of every age sitting in deck chairs observing the sociable scene. Some were dangling feet in the steamy froth, others were plunged up to their necks in the pool—faces displaying that slightly bemused, soporific calm—off in a water world of their own.

The rooms at Nance's are nothing to rave about, but the view from them is. The second-floor rooms, sheltered by a long porch, look out over the valley and glider field immediately adjacent—a green expanse of fields leading to rows of grapevines. The vineyards stretching beyond blanket the hills with a crazy-quilt pattern, the rows oriented first one way and then another in regular patches.

On sunny afternoons the upper balcony hosts groups of people sitting together soaking up the rays, drinking wine, playing guitars and looking at the view. A most pleasant, informal place.

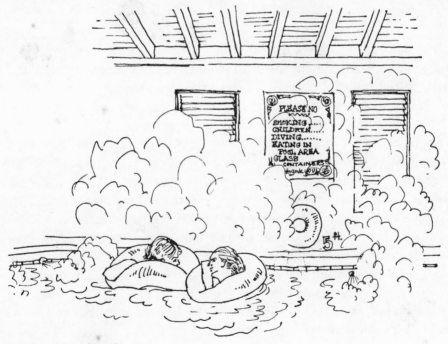

Indoor hot mineral pool,
Nance's Hot Springs, Calistoga

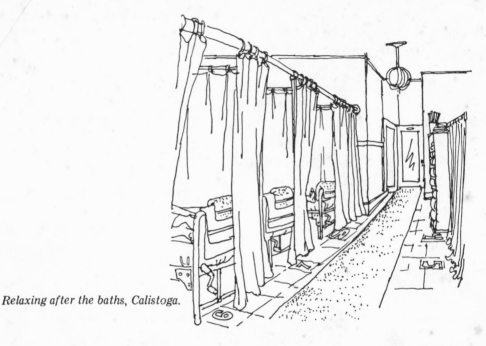

Relaxing after the baths, Calistoga.

The motel rooms are equipped with kitchens, utensils and dishes, television, air conditioning and access to the long sunny balcony which runs the length of the motel. Located on Lincoln Avenue, the main street of Calistoga, Nance's is within easy walking distance of several cafes and restaurants, a stroll away from Dr. Wilkerson's and Pacheteau's spas.

The management of Nance's swears by the healing quality of the volcanic-ash mud baths, and as did their forebearers who established spas here in the 1800s, they recognize the mud and mineral waters as Nature's remedy for rheumatism, neuritis, arthritis and various nerve and muscular ailments. This, of course, is no joke. Many medical specialists today recommend hot water treatments and relaxation for these and other stress-related disorders. Frankly, we prefer to take our cure in the hot water. But clearly the mud, a source of deep heat penetration that in turn increases blood circulation, is a therapy favored by scores of people who come here yearly.

For simple relaxation, in addition to the hot mud, try hot sulphur and steam baths followed by a blanket sweat and a cool shower. Massage by well-trained masseurs on the men's side and masseuses in the women's quarters is available.

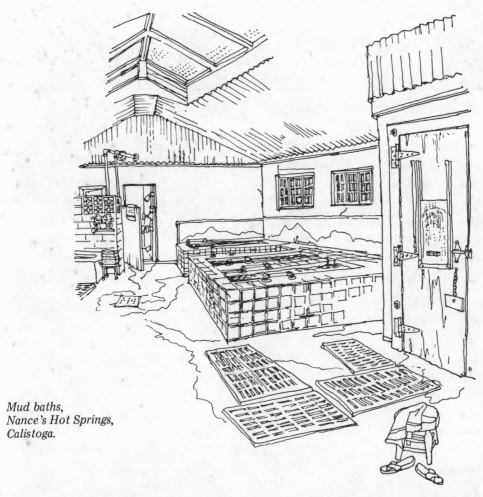

Mud baths,
Nance's Hot Springs,
Calistoga.

NANCE'S HOT SPRINGS, 1614 Lincoln Avenue, Calistoga, California 94515. Telephone: (707) 942-6211. Accommodations: air-conditioned rooms with kitchenettes; private baths; single and double beds; no telephones; cable television. Rates: $18 single, $20 double. No meal service. Reservations recommended. No children under 12. No pets. Cards: BA, MC, VISA. Open all year.

Spa facilities: Hot mineral pool with Jacuzzi jets, no charge; volcanic mud bath, mineral bath, steam room and blanket sweat, massage, $18; lower rates for other combinations of service from $6. Bathing suits required in communal pools; suits optional in separate men's and women's quarters.

PACHETEAU'S HOT SPRINGS
Calistoga

Ah! Fantastic, fumarolic Pacheteau's. The most informal, richest in history, least altered, most carefully laid out of all the Calistoga spas. And the most beautiful view of Calistoga is gained by climbing the hills back of Pacheteau's. Immediately beneath your feet are turquoise-blue holding tanks of hot mineral water, glistening in the sun, and even on the hottest day raising steamy puffs to the open sky. Spectacular hissing, geyser-like sprays escape from mineral-encrusted valves sitting right atop the earth. Just beyond is the clear blue expanse of the hot Olympic-size pool for which Pacheteau's is famous. And still beyond, laid out like the old pictures in history books, are the drives and grounds of the bathhouse and cabins of what was Calistoga's

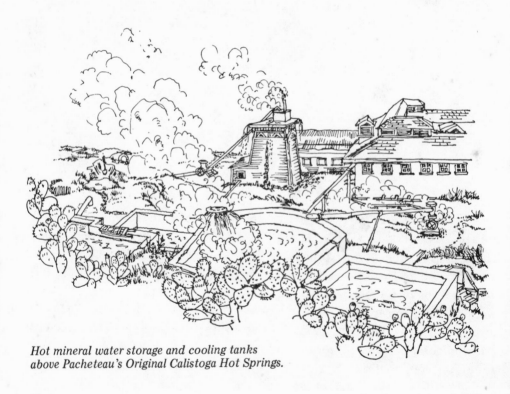

Hot mineral water storage and cooling tanks
above Pacheteau's Original Calistoga Hot Springs.

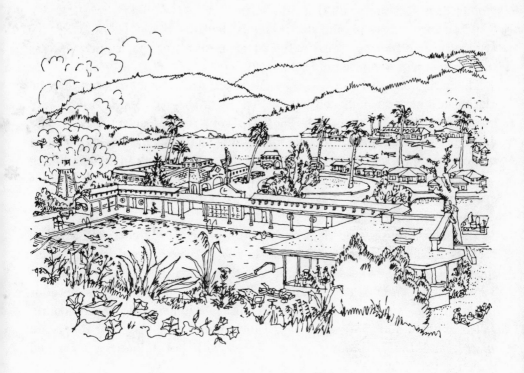

first spa—in 1862, the grandest spa in the West, visited by the rich, famous and talented. In 1880 Robert Louis Stevenson, occupied one of the cottages (now on view downtown in Calistoga as an historic monument), and wrote parts of *Silverado Squatters* on the spa grounds.

Calistoga was the dream of one Sam Brannan, colorful, charismatic California pioneer, who made a fortune in the state's gold fields and who christened the town of Calistoga by a slip of the tongue. Sam's dream was to make his spa as famed as the Saratoga Hot Springs of New York. One evening at a party he was telling his friends and family why he was pouring a fortune into hot water and a wilderness. With his usual impetuosity and energy he exclaimed, "I will make this place the Calistoga of Sarafonia!" And so it is.

Today the pride of Pacheteau's is the huge, outdoor swimming pool that shimmers aquamarine in the valley sun; in the cooler mornings and on cloudy days soft mists rise from the surface as you swim in the warm water. Children love this pool, and on weekends the surrounding lawns and decks are merry with families from the town and guests at the spa. You may picnic on the lawn with the birds and squirrels.

The bathhouses at Pacheteau's are clean, but funky. One imagines that the blackened, mineral-encrusted pipes that skirt the bathhouse floors were installed by Brannan's workers. The old clawed-foot porcelain soaking tubs are kept whistling clean. The wooden floors and walls have been scrubbed over the years to a soft, grey sheen. Even the exotic algae and lichen peeking out between the wallboards of the steam room seem to have found this comfortable niche long ago. A mud bath at Pacheteau's is *really* getting down to basics.

The cabins are situated right on the edge of the flat, greensward reserved for glider landings. The best bargain in town, these three-room and four-room cottages line the same gentle curve of drive that circled the spa in 1860. Large, comfortably padded redwood furniture surrounds outdoor tables on the lawn of each cabin. The cottage kitchens are 1930s modern, fully equipped and spotlessly clean. The furnishings of the other rooms are simple, and the bathrooms are mini-spas with hot sulphur water piped directly in.

Restored cottage, circa 1860, from Sam Brannan's original Calistoga hot springs, now a private home.

The old, traditional mud and steam rooms,
Pacheteau's Hot Springs, Calistoga.

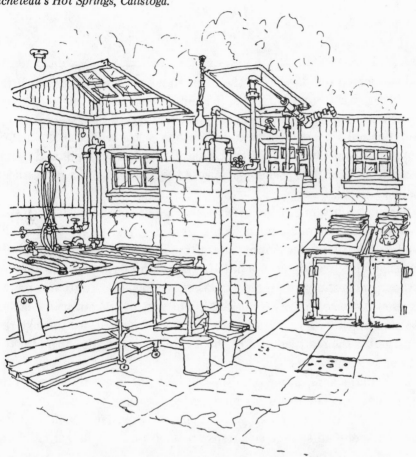

PACHETEAU'S ORIGINAL CALISTOGA HOT SPRINGS, 1712 Lincoln Avenue, Calistoga, California 94515. Telephone: (707) 942-5589. Accommodations: housekeeping cabins with fully equipped kitchens; private baths; twin and double beds; no telephones; extra charge for television. Rates: $20, plus $10 for each extra person. No meal service. Reservations recommended. Children welcome. No pets. Cards: BA, MC, VISA. Open all year.
Spa facilities: swimming pool, $2.50; steam cabinet, blanket sweat, tub with sulphur steam bath $6, with mud bath $7.50; massage and shower $10. Bathing suits required in outdoor pool; suits optional in separate men's and women's quarters.

ROMAN SPA
Calistoga

Roman Spa, located one block off the main street of Calistoga, differs little from the other spas in town. That is, it is unpretentious, prosperous, clean and comfortable, and blessed with an abundance of hot, mineral water.

Roman Spa, like most of the old Calistoga spas, is in the process of remodeling. Built on the site of historic Piner Lodge, some rooms and cabins still remain from the 1920s, side-by-side with the new California-style stucco motel units.

The charming courtyard of the old Piner Lodge has been transformed into a quiet expanse of hot pools open to the wind, sky and lovely light of the Napa Valley. We spent one happy late afternoon here, wrapped in warm robes and sipping burgundy after a hot afternoon's hike through the hills. As the afternoon moves toward evening and the air cools, the crowd around the pool becomes more sociable. People slip in and out of the hot water, steam now rises high into the air. The late afternoon sun slants down through the palm trees, across the red-tiled roof of the main building; birds chirp over the faint hum of swirling waters.

The spa facilities here, other than the outdoor pools, are rather small by Calistoga standards. There are no mud baths, for example. But there are sauna units, and massage and physical therapy is available. Children are welcome, but there are some restrictions on pool use for younger children.

ROMAN SPA, 1300 Washington Street, Calistoga, California 94515. Telephone: (707) 942-4441. Accommodations: rooms; single, double, queen-size beds; no telephones; television; some fully equipped kitchens, some cooktop units. Rates: from $18 in original lodge rooms; from $28 in new units; $38 for four in two-bedroom units. No meal service. Reservations recommended. Children welcome. Some pets allowed by special request. Cards: BA, MC. Open all year.

Spa facilities: hot mineral pool, Jacuzzi, sauna, no charge to overnight guests; massage and physical therapy, $15 to $23 per hour.

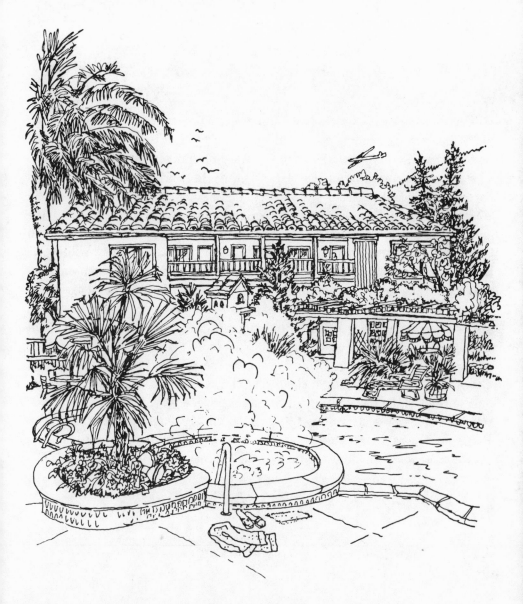

Hot pools in the courtyard, Roman Spa, Calistoga.

WILBUR HOT SPRINGS
Wilbur Springs, Colusa County

Wilbur Hot Springs is a secluded country spa 20 miles from the nearest town in the heart of the rolling coastal hills of California. It is 120 miles northeast of San Francisco; follow the map to the junction of Highways 16 and 20 where you follow the sign that says "Wilbur Hot Springs" onto a dirt road cut into the hillside.

The road hangs above a small, perfectly proportioned valley, and the experience of Wilbur begins with this drive. A rushing stream cuts through the valley, the same stream that flows beneath the bathhouse of Wilbur. As the road crosses the stream over an arched silver bridge, one often encounters the strong smell of sulphur. For newcomers this may be a barrier to cross, for old timers it evokes the pleasures to come. The rocks of the stream are covered with heavy deposits of minerals, and little steamy rivulets cut through the grassy meadows.

Through a wooden gate you drive into the private property of Wilbur. Down the lane is an old barn sheltering chickens, goats and pigs, and rising on the right is the old Wilbur Hot Springs Lodge, a grey, three-storied stucco structure still in use after 60 years. Located on 240 acres of countryside, this lodge once was the center of cabins, barns, bathhouses and gardens of a much larger spa popular at the turn of the century.

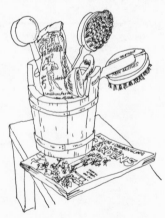

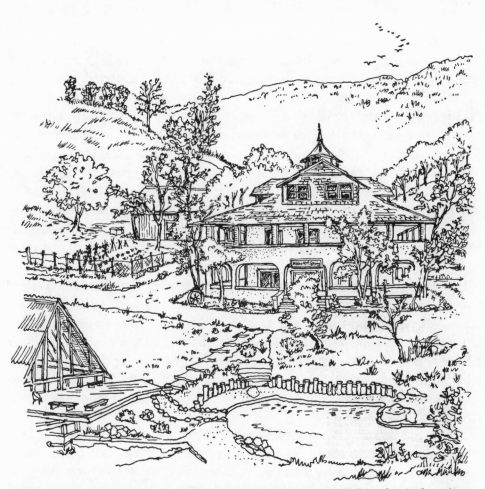

The lodge and grounds have been lovingly restored by the industrious group of people who live year round at Wilbur. Led by R. L. Miller, Ph.D., the staff of Wilbur is devoted to preserving the facilities as a health sanctuary and restful retreat for their guests. Richard Miller and the Wilbur staff recently organized an impressive and successful campaign to save the hot springs on their land from geothermal exploration and development on the grounds that the springs and environs are valuable for therapeutic, medical, cultural and historic reasons. Wilbur Hot Springs is now eligible to be listed on the National Register as a historic landmark.

Leave your car in the designated area, walk back to the lodge and check in at the desk. Someone will show you where to place your bedding if you are staying all night, and give you a tour of the kitchen and grounds.

Wilbur is a retreat for everyone of all ages, and most of the guests are families and groups who bring their children along. This is one of the few places where children are welcome in the baths, under supervision of course.

Across the road from the lodge is the spacious new bathhouse. Built of rustic redwood and glass, it cantilevers over the stream bed and overlooks the countryside. Local custom here allows either nude bathing or suits. You may leave your clothes outside the bathhouse and proceed nude, as many do, or you may change clothes in your lodge quarters and cross the road to the baths in kimono and zoris.

The baths here are a delight. As you enter the bathhouse, rows of tubs complete with bobbing bodies, are spread out before you. Choose your temperature! The first tub to try is the third one in from the door—a conservative 95 degrees. Temperature in the other tubs rises gradually to 120 degrees so you have a choice of four temperatures. The tubs are separated from one another by plank decks suitable for lounging and cooling; pegs are handy for robes and towels, although it's OK to drop them on the decks.

Ease into the 95-degree tub and study the Wilbur routine. Bathers move back and forth from pool to pool. Some take a cold-water shower inside the bathhouse and return to the hot pools. Some go outside to the ice-cold swimming pool between hot-tub dips. Others soak awhile and lounge awhile. Some meditate.

You will be spending your indoor time at Wilbur in this bathhouse or in the lodge. Here we have nested comfortably in a private room upstairs, as well as in sleeping bags on a veranda that borders the hotel on three sides.

Our favorite room at the lodge is the kitchen, especially at meal time when everyone is rubbing elbows and talking together animatedly as they prepare their food. It's difficult not to get into the spirit of warmth and hospitality that prevails at mealtime and characterizes one's whole stay at Wilbur. Bring with you to Wilbur whatever you will need in the way of towels, sheets, food or drink. There are no stores on the grounds and remember you are 20 miles from the nearest town. There is refrigerator space for you in the kitchen. Stove, cooking ware, plates and cutlery are provided.

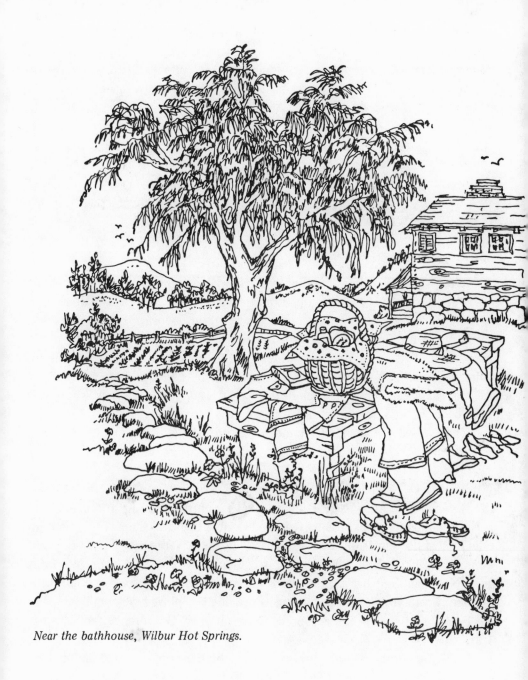

Near the bathhouse, Wilbur Hot Springs.

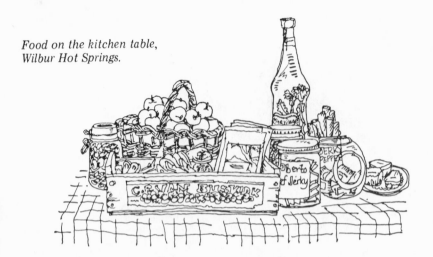

Food on the kitchen table,
Wilbur Hot Springs.

Massage is available by appointment for one-half hour or one hour. When we were there, we had a skilled masseuse, whose table was set up in a secluded spot of the veranda. The Wilbur body work-massage is a deep massage, combining shiatsu and pressure point massage with lighter relaxation work. The masseuse may direct you to breathe deeply from time to time, as breathing exercises accompany the massage. This is not a light, sensual massage, nor it is a painful process. But you definitely know you have been worked on when it's over.

Yoga classes are available some weekends, taught by Jay De Roy, an experienced teacher and yogi disciple.

WILBUR HOT SPRINGS, Wilbur Springs, California 95987. Telephone: (916) 473-2306. Accommodations: private rooms and group rooms; private baths and shared baths; bunk, twin and double beds; no linens furnished; no telephones; no television. Rates: $16 per person, Wednesday, Thursday and Sunday; $21 to $32 per person, weekends; weekly and monthly rates available, including barter and work exchange. Meals cooked in communal kitchen; bring your own food, utensils provided. Children welcome. No pets. No credit cards or checks accepted. Open all year. Conference facilities for 100 available.

Spa facilities: hot natural spring water tubs; ice-cold, spring-fed outdoor swimming pool; massage; yoga classes; $5 for day use; no charge for overnight guests. Bathing suits optional.

ORR HOT SPRINGS
Ukiah, Mendocino County

We've known hot-spring devotees who will pursue rumors of mineral baths down country roads, across state lines and into uncharted mountains; those who soak only in hot mineral waters in natural pools or once removed into pond or tub. Orr Hot Springs is their spa.

Orr is nestled in a rustic setting deep in the coastal hills of Mendocino County, 14 miles west of Highway 101 just north of Ukiah. The accommodations are primitive, even by California country-spa standards; cabins and campsites are grouped in quiet, wooded seclusion among various large containers that trap the continuous flow of hot water right from the earth.

With little effort of the imagination, you are back in the 1880s, one of the hardy pioneers who has made his way by stagecoach, horse and foot to the curative waters of the California mountains. Folks go here for the calm of the countryside, for a retreat. And the hospitable bright people who run Orr intend just that: "You'll find these waters very relaxing for your body and your soul."

The style of Orr is informal. The group that lives here and operates the springs is composed of friendly people who welcome you immediately upon arrival. Their lodge is open for those who wish to lounge about inside or use the kitchen to do their own cooking.

Hot, natural spring water flows into several old-fashioned bathtubs, but Orr management has just installed a new, large redwood hot tub that holds eight comfortably. It may replace the old communal corrugated metal tub nearby as a favorite soak of ours. There is also a large, cold-water swimming pool fed by mineral spring water.

You may use all the facilities at Orr for a day, or you may stay longer sleeping in your own bedroll, in cabins or in the lounge. If you choose to camp-out in the little woods past the pool, there are small cleared areas there for pitching a tent or putting down your sleeping bag. The stars at night are right on top of you. The little redwood cabins are more private, of course, with beds and baths. And in the lodge is a large loft where you can roll out your sleeping bag on Japanese mats along with other mosquito-haters.

While at Orr, plan some strolls around the countryside or a longer hike in the hills of Mendocino County; they are enchanting and intimate and the climate is cool and invigorating at all times. The stands of oak and evergreen around Orr spa are ancient, beautiful, and the months of April to November are particularly excellent for camping and hiking.

In the summer you may buy three meals a day at the lodge. Breakfast is hearty with eggs, fruit, cereal, a choice of delicious teas and coffee; lunch is sandwiches only, and the dinners are more elaborate and vegetarian.

Children and pets are welcome; bring your own towels, bathing suits, and other accoutrements you would pack for a day in the woods.

ORR HOT SPRINGS, Star Route 1, Box 7, Orr Springs Road, Ukiah, California 95482. Telephone: (707) 462-6277. Accommodations: cabins with single and double beds; campsites; shared baths; no telephones; no television. Rates: $8 to $9 outdoor/indoor camping; $15 for cabin, plus $10 for each additional person. Breakfast, lunch and dinner served at lodge. Reservations advised. Children and pets welcome. No credit cards. Open all year.
Spa facilities: communal hot tubs, large swimming pool; $3.50 per day for use of all facilities, including the kitchen; no charge for overnight guests. Bathing suits optional in hot tubs.

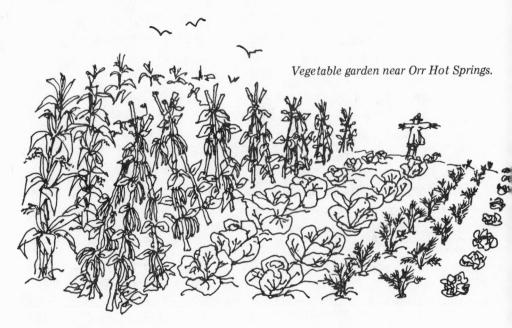

Vegetable garden near Orr Hot Springs.

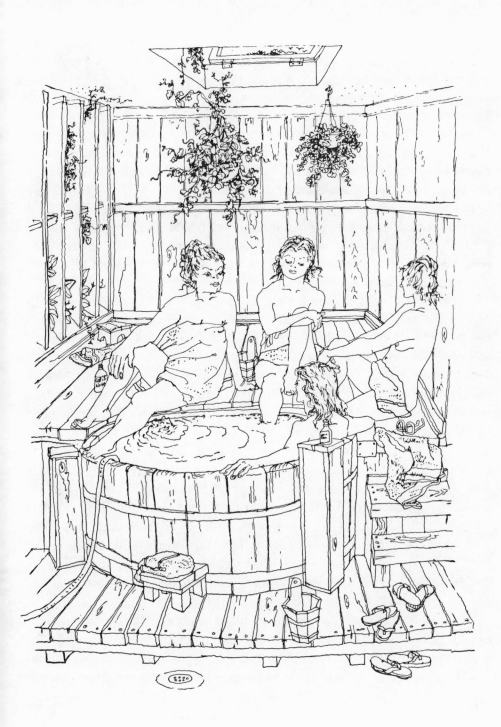

CAMPBELL HOT SPRINGS
Sierraville, Sierra County

Campbell Hot Springs is located in the most spectacular of natural settings. High in the Sierras, nestled at the foot of a forested mountain, the front porch of the old white wooden hotel looks out for miles over a fertile mountain valley to the peaks beyond.

In summer, the valley shimmers in heat at midday; one is grateful to be in the shade of tall pines which surround the hotel. In winter, the valley is a flat field of snow, beckoning cross-country skiers away from the hot tubs and into the countryside. In any season, the night sky is immense and filled with diamond-bright stars.

Since 1850, Campbell Hot Springs has been known as a place to take the waters; the present hotel was built in 1909. There have been few changes in the building or its view down over the valley since that time. The sense of space, of seclusion, of rustic country living are still intact.

The hotel and hot springs are now owned and operated by a friendly group of individuals who live at Campbell as a community year round. In addition to operating Campbell as a hotel and spa, they offer seminars on topics as diverse as "Investment and Money" and "Loving Relationships." They urge you to "give yourself a vacation in the country, with as many friends as you want to create. People who appreciate natural hot springs are special people, and basically we have two kinds of guests. Those who prefer their privacy and there is lots of room to be alone here, and those who are more gregarious and like company to be with ... either friends they bring with them or the community that is here at Campbell. We welcome all kinds." We looked in on some of the classes offered at the resort by community members, and we also spent time sticking to our own country routine, using their accommodations and hot tubs.

Facilities at Campbell Hot Spring include the hotel with accommodations for 20 people. Additional rooms are available in another hotel owned by the community located in Sierraville, a mile away. Both hotels are open year round and many people use them as a center for snow sports—cross-country

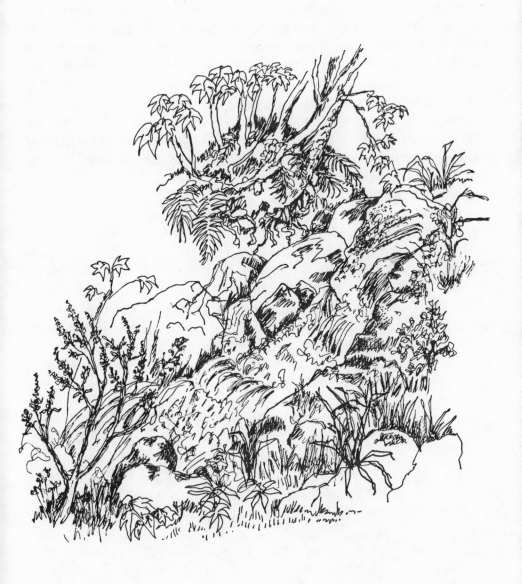

Mountain waterfall, northern California.

skiing, backpacking, skiing at nearby Lake Tahoe, snowshoeing and ice skating. The roads are cleared throughout the winter by daily snowplow.

The hot tubs here are small by other spa standards; two rock-lined tubs each hold about eight people at a time comfortably. The tubs require a walk of about one-half mile from the hotel. The water is hot enough, and plentiful, and when we visited the management had built a new wooden bathhouse surrounding the tubs.

There is another mineral pool adjoining the hotel filled with cool natural mineral water. It is lined round with a sundeck and neat rows of wooden bath stalls that appear to be part of the original spa facilities—quaint, painted white with louvered wood doors from which one expects a woman to emerge dressed in black wool bloomers and tank top.

Meals may be taken in the hotel restaurant at Campbell Hot Springs. If you choose, you may bring your own food and prepare meals in the large community kitchen. Nearby Sierraville has several country cafes and bars.

CAMPBELL HOT SPRINGS, P.O. Box 38, Sierraville, California 96126. Telephone: (916) 994-3318. Accommodations: hotel rooms; shared bath; single and double beds; no telephones; no television. Rates: $15 single, $22.50 double, lunch and dinner included. Reservations recommended. Children welcome. No pets. No credit cards accepted. Open all year.
Spa facilities: natural, rock-lined hot tubs, natural mineral-water swimming pool, $5 per day for all facilities. Bathing suits optional in hot tubs.

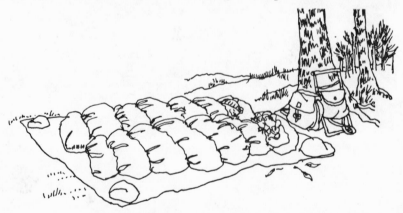

Sleeping under the stars near Campbell Hot Springs.

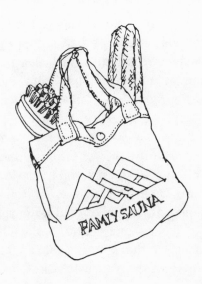

FAMILY SAUNA SHOP
San Francisco

Sonja Lillvik, president of the Family Sauna Shop, has taken enormous pains to re-create an authentic sauna in San Francisco. She also has clearly established her two shops as places for the family and the community—as she had known them to be when growing up in the Finnish community of Vinland, a small town in New Jersey. Both shops reflect her painstaking care, not only in the design and atmosphere of the facilities, but in her gentle insistence that we learn to appreciate "how does a sauna mean" rather than going in with a competitive or grin-and-bear-it attitude.

Sonja and her staff believe a sauna should give you time to be "still and quiet," with a total effect of making you feel "unbelievably clean, undeniably relaxed, but energized to go on." To this end, she has prepared "Some Hints and Suggestions for Experimentation as You Find Your Own 'Best Way' to Sauna." It is worth reading, and we would encourage you to begin your sojourn into the land of hot tub and sauna with this background. Even if you are an "old-hand" we think you would find Sonja's way of approaching the sauna in Finnish tradition a pleasant discovery.

Sonja suggests that you start your sauna on the top bench (the hottest spot in the sauna room) and, when you begin to perspire, ladle just a *little* cold water onto the heater rocks until you feel a rush of moist air. This process can be repeated at intervals. When your face feels warm, dip a washcloth in cold water and dampen your entire face and neck. Until you find your own "best way," move back and forth from upper to lower benches—even into the dressing area outside for a few minutes' break. At the end of the half-hour, move to the shower area, fill the bucket provided with soapy water and sit on the stool, preferably having a friend or family member scrub you down from head to toe. At this point, rinse off well under the shower, finishing with a cool or cold water spray.

For the second half of your sauna period, Sonja advises that you simply stretch out on the bench in the dressing room and close your eyes to everything. Family Sauna provides you with a soft, cotton wrap-around and scuffs and there is a buzzer in your room to ring for a juice. Finally, Sonja recommends that you take either a hot tub *or* a sauna, but not both on the same day.

The atmosphere at both locations exudes gentleness and simplicity, and the staff is particularly warm and helpful. We heartily recommend Family Sauna as a starting place for those who are about to embark on this wonderful new-old way to unwind and restore inner serenity.

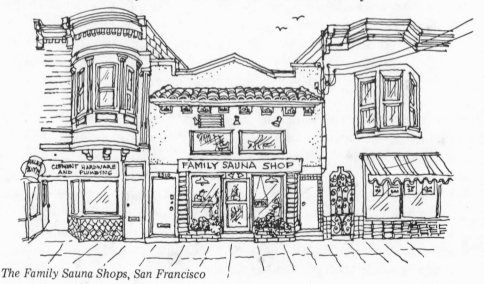

The Family Sauna Shops, San Francisco

Sundeck, Family Sauna on 20th Avenue, San Francisco.

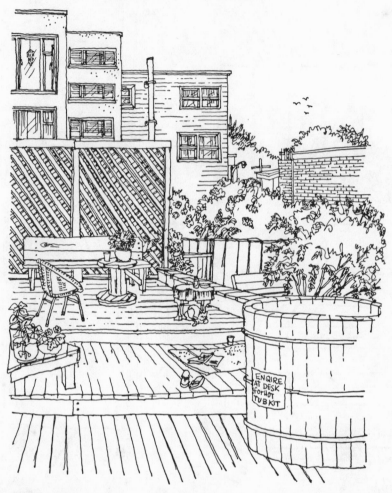

The Shop on 20th Avenue

This facility has four cedar and redwood saunas; three are fairly large and one is smaller. There is no hot tub. Massage is scheduled by appointment. In the back of the Family Sauna, tucked into this quiet neighborhood, is a small deck with benches and tables; you can wander out here in your wrap-around and scuffs and stretch out in the sun on those days when San Francisco weather is feeling generous.

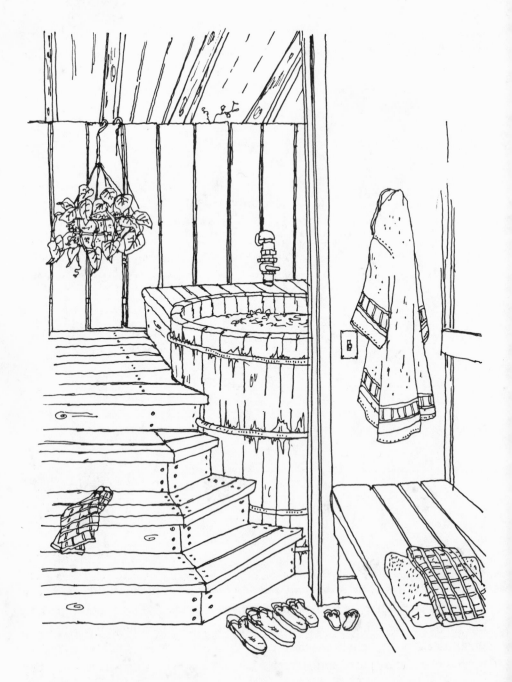

Hot tub room, Family Sauna on Clement Street, San Francisco.

The Shop on Clement Street

Clement Street has saunas as well as two hot tubs. One tub is small and cozily housed in redwood; hanging plants and sunlight flickering in through the beams make you forget you are on a busy San Francisco street. The other, just finished, is a large plastic tub that holds four or five. Each tub room has its own outer dressing-room area with towels, floor mat, mirror and electrical outlet (for a hair dryer you can obtain from the desk). Perrier water or juice will be brought to you, should you want to relax with a cold drink when you finish. The hot tub room has an open shower area with bucket, back-scrubber, liquid soap and wooden stool.

Each sauna opens onto two separate dressing rooms. If one group is not using both rooms, the entry and exit from sauna to dressing area is carefully orchestrated by the desk so that while you are on your resting half-hour, another guest can enter the sauna. Again, you will find a wooden stool and scrub brush near the sauna room shower, and a bucket and ladle for pouring water over the rocks. The staff will put a plastic pool in the sauna room for children so that they can splash in cooler water at floor level where the heat is less intense. (It goes without saying that children must be with adults.)

There is no outside deck here, but a charming loft over the reception area looks out on busy Clement Street. Magazines and games are there for your use—a lovely place to relax after your sauna or tub. Massage is offered at both shops and massage classes are scheduled at Clement Street. Lotions and potions are sold at the counter.

The Family Sauna Shop has been described as "the most authentic sauna in town" by the *San Francisco Chronicle,* and a "one-hour vacation" by Caroline Mufford writing for *Business Monthly's* profile of Sonja Lillvik in "Enterprising Women." We can attest to the truth of both statements.

FAMILY SAUNA SHOP, 1208 20th Avenue, San Francisco, California 94122. Telephone: (415) 681-3600. 2308 Clement Street, San Francisco, California 94121. Telephone: (415) 221-2208. No overnight accommodations. No meal service. No reservations, except for massage. Cards: BA, MC. Open 12 to 10; 20th Avenue shop closed Tuesday; Clement Street shop closed Monday.

Spa facilities: sauna, $3.50; hot tubs, $3.50 to $4; massage, $15 per hour, $8 for one-half hour.

GRAND CENTRAL SAUNA & HOT TUB
San Francisco

Grand Central Sauna changed owners in 1976 and at this writing branch facilities are in blueprint stages for Berkeley, Mountain View and Seattle. A spiffy clean, cheerful and beautifully maintained spa, its new owners are obviously proud of their facility and determined to maintain high-quality standards. You feel so good from the moment you walk into the bright blue, green and white lobby, that you are ready to buy a Grand Central T-shirt even before you see the fantastic tub/sauna room that is to be yours for an hour or more of solid relaxation.

Manager Roger Dorfman escorts newcomers to their spa room and points out its many fine features as if conducting a house tour. There are 26 private, self-contained tub/sauna rooms, each housing a lovely redwood hot tub with a Jacuzzi operated by wall switch, a tiled but open shower area, a closeted redwood sauna, a double mattress at tub height, a clothes/towel rack, a telephone and a large wall clock. Light switches are equipped with a dimmer, and a variety of music, from 1940s favorites to soft rock, is piped into each room. Tub water is maintained at approximately 105 degrees and temperature in the sauna room hovers around 185 degrees—which is *hot;* do not overdo it.

Once your facility has been shown to you, and the procedure explained, you are left to your enjoyment until the front desk rings—10 minutes before the hour is up. If you decide to remain an extra half hour, you can simply tell the desk at that time. You can also ring the desk for juice.

Grand Central invites singles, couples and families, (one large hot tub room holds six and opens to an adjoining room for a group of 12) but their clientele is mostly couples. The facility has been designed for maximum privacy and comfort, and is conscientiously cared for; water chlorination and pH is checked four times daily, for example. The owners have resisted all outside attempts to commercialize their interior. They do not ever intend to clutter up their lobby with advertisements and pictures, and the only "commodities" sold are their Grand Central T-shirts and juices. They are also responsible about alcohol use—it is not allowed. Anyone who has been

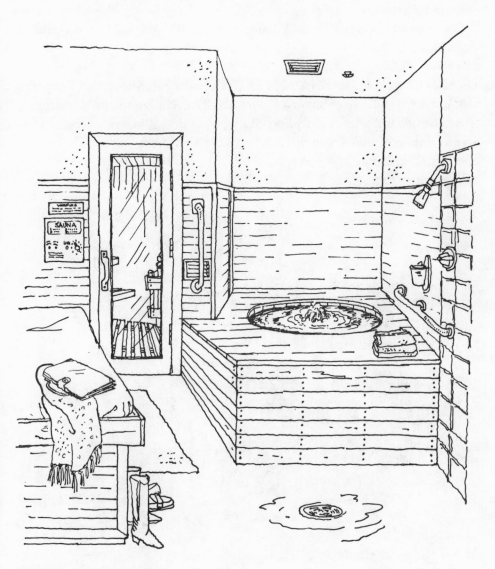

Hot tub, massage and sauna room.
Grand Central Sauna and Hot Tub, San Francisco.

drinking is discouraged from using the spa and, if obviously inebriated, is not permitted to stay.

No reservations are accepted. Mondays and Tuesdays are generally slower than the rest of the week. The longest wait, we were told, is one hour or an hour and a half on a busy evening.

Overheard chuckle: If Family Saunas are the FM of spas, Grand Central is the AM.

GRAND CENTRAL SAUNA AND HOT TUB, 15 Fell Street, San Francisco, California 94102. Telephone: (415) 431-1370. No overnight accommodations. No meal service; fruit juices available. Reservations not accepted. No credit cards accepted. Open daily, 11 to midnight.

Spa facilities: sauna and hot tubs, $4.25 to $4.50 per person; minimum of two persons after 5 p.m.

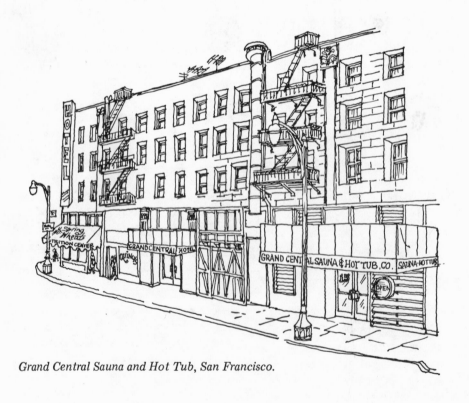

Grand Central Sauna and Hot Tub, San Francisco.

KABUKI HOT SPRING
San Francisco

Kabuki Hot Spring has become justifiably famous for its unprecedented spa experience, as well as for its fabulous equipment and service. And there is a truly novel feature here that caused a friend to earnestly entreat, "Come with me right now. You will not *believe* this.": A Japanese shiatsu expert gives an outstanding massage that leaves you as relaxed as you are ever likely to feel.

Located in Japan Center on bustling Geary Boulevard, Kabuki Hot Spring has the feeling of present-day Tokyo where the traditional is dressed in modern garb. You will discern details here that are similar to the hot baths of quiet Japanese country inns.

At first glance the building itself, with its large plate-glass doors and lobby, seems like a well-designed and well-appointed office building, exuding calm efficiency and understated elegance. Traditional Japanese music filters through the lobby where a receptionist waits to serve you and to call out the attendant who will greet you in the lobby and lead you to the men's or women's quarters. The quality of service is quite high; you will be given every personal attention.

Once past the lobby, however, a traditional Japanese bathhouse emerges, in feeling if not in decor. If you are a woman, your attendant—a massaji-shi —remains with you from the time you enter until the time you leave. If you are a man, she will usher you to the men's quarters, reappear from time to time with towels and offers of service, and will give you a massage. Kabuki Hot Spring offers separate and distinct services for men and women; not only in the attendance of the massaji-shi, but in the design of the facilities, the type of services and the prices.

Women's Facilities

All of the following services, with the exception of the sauna, take place in a single, private room equipped with a dressing table, closet, massage table on one side and a "wet area" a few stairs away. The attendant ushers, leads and directs you through each step of the process. Massaji-shis, fresh from two to four years of massage schooling in Japan, speak little English. But we found that no barrier to communication, for our attendant was smiling and happy to engage in all sorts of sign language, body language and simple exchanges such as "too hot," "ouch," and "oh wow."

As soon as you are in your room and have disrobed, the massaji-shi will direct you to the shower. There is a stool in the shower area, and she may tell you to sit down while she scrubs your back with a loufa, a long cylindrical sponge with a pleasantly rough surface. When you are thoroughly rinsed, you will be directed to the hot tub and, once comfortably immersed, she may leave you for a short interval of time, returning when it is time to move on to a steam bath or sauna.

You may choose next a steam bath, sauna or both, and the massaji-shi will help regulate the steam for you and then wrap you in a sheet for your short walk down a carpeted hallway to the sauna room. These are cedar-lined and reflect the same simple elegance that you see and feel throughout Kabuki. Again, you will be left to soak up the heat, assured that your attendant will re-appear when it is time to continue on to the next phase.

Now you are ready for the massage. Wrapped again in your sheet and ushered back to your private room, you are in for an unforgettable experience—the Japanese shiatsu massage. Shiatsu is distinctly different from other massage techniques, involving deep finger pressure and tissue kneading of selected tension points all over the body. Your attendant is an expert at it, and while it takes approximately 30 minutes in physical time, your body will feel light years removed from its former state.

For the novice, traditional shiatsu can be somewhat painful and, if you have not spoken up at the first pressure point, do not hesitate to let the massaji-shi know if pain begins to overtake pleasure. The total experience of this massage should be one of sheer delight.

Bring only yourself and a change of clothing if you wish to Kabuki. From the time you hang up your street clothes, you will be nude or moving about in a towel or sheet wrap. You will not encounter others, however, except your massaji-shi. A tray of beauty aids will be in the dressing room area, and towels, sheets, soaps are provided.

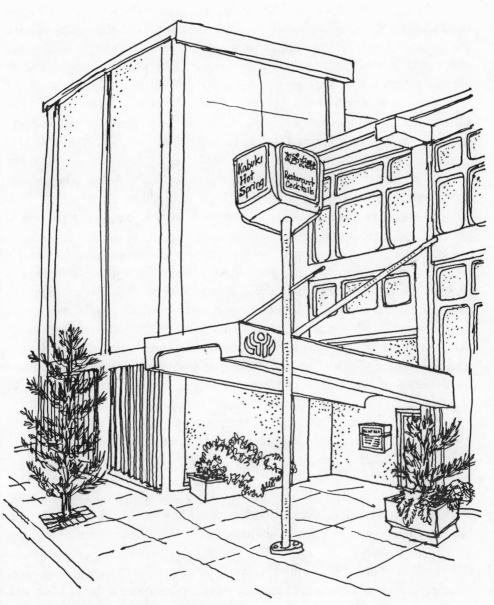

Kabuki Hot Spring entrance, San Francisco.

Men's Facilities

The men's quarters at Kabuki Hot Spring are remarkable for their functional design and restful ambience. The spa is only five years old and equipped with the latest in bath and gym appliances. The large central "wet room" is the epitome of spa efficiency at its most attractive—a wealth of tile, sparkling chrome and glass shares space with warm wood benches, saunas and stacks of soft white towels and sheets. You are free to take the waters from steam bath to cold, needle-spray showers, moving at your own pace and concentrating on your own needs and feeling of well-being.

One huge tiled hot tub—used communally—is in the center of the room which also houses a cold tub, showers, steam baths and sauna. The Jacuzzi runs constantly, and there is no time limit imposed on your soak. "Self-service" steam cabinets line one of the walls of this big room; the use is optional and there is again no time limit imposed.

Easily the largest sauna room we have seen covers one wall of the men's area. You enter through sliding glass doors; in fact, the whole wall facing the room is glass. There are three levels of redwood benches. No time limit is imposed, but 15 minutes is the suggested time to spend at 145 degrees.

Should you wish a massage, your name will be called on a loudspeaker in the communal tub room when your reservation time approaches. The massage is Japanese shiatsu, identical to that in the women's quarters. You will leave the communal area and enter a large, carpeted room containing couches, exercise equipment and massage tables. The massaji-shi will greet you at the door and show you to the massage table; after the 30-minute massage, you will remain on the table for a 15-minute rest.

KABUKI HOT SPRING, 1750 Geary Boulevard, San Francisco, California 94115. Telephone: (415) 922-6000. No overnight accommodations. No meal service. Reservations required. Children not allowed. No pets. Cards: BA, MC. Open all year; women's facilities, 12 to 7:30 daily; men's facilities, 11:30 to 10 daily.

Spa facilities: hot tubs, steam cabinets, Jacuzzi, sauna, massage, gym. Rates: women, $20 for all services and massage; men, $5 for baths only, $17 for bath and massage. Nudity or towel wrap optional in separate men's and women's quarters.

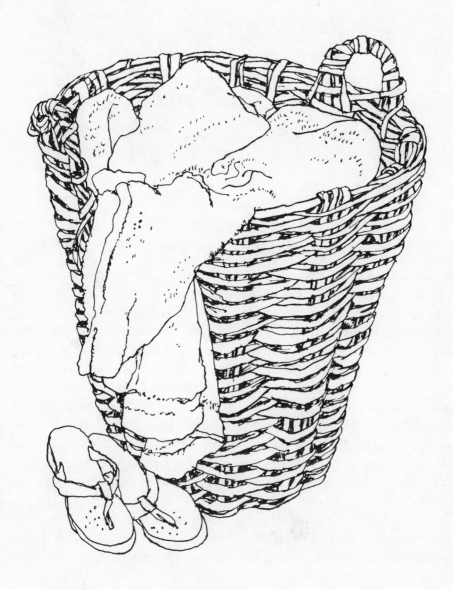

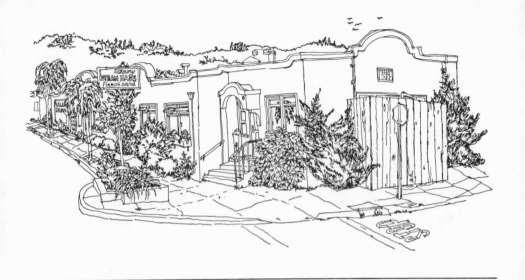

ALBANY SAUNA
Albany, Alameda County

Albany Sauna is located on the main street of the small, thriving Bay Area town from which it takes its name. The surrounding shops, post office, grocery stores, shade trees and sidewalk parking make for a neighborly, friendly atmosphere. This same comfortable feeling follows you into Albany Sauna—right up to the front desk where you are greeted by one of the young owners/managers of this favorite of East Bay watering holes.

The owners moved here four years ago from the East Coast, to escape the pressures of top jobs and the stresses of urban crowding. Taking over an established and rather formal Finnish sauna, they created a warm, relaxed atmosphere for all ages, increasing the popularity of this sauna until lines began to stretch out the door on weekends. Book in advance or expect a wait most days.

Albany Sauna's facilities are spartan, no-nonsense, small and clean. Help and assistance are available for the asking, but you are expected to fit yourself into the calm, simple routines of the place—moving quietly from steam room to massage room.

Occupying a plain, stucco building, with few internal frills, this is a typical urban bathhouse. The building has been modified on the interior to hold its

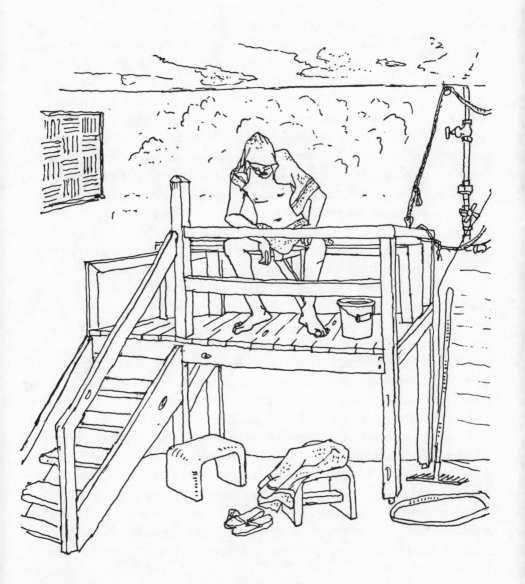

Traditional Finnish steam room, Albany Sauna, Albany.

large central oven and big wooden hot tubs. Despite its plainness, you will enjoy the efficient service, the neighborhood atmosphere and the experience of hot steam from one of the few remaining Finnish saunas.

About this Finnish sauna: Sauna rooms are arranged around an enormous centrally located oven and each is approached through a private dressing room. A bell timer is provided to remind you when to leave the sauna; an attendant will base the time you should stay on your stated experience with saunas. Instructions for adjusting the oven heat are printed on a card on the wall and should be read immediately upon entering the sauna. These wet-heat sauna rooms are quite ample in size, plain, with wooden stairs leading up to a high bench for maximum heat. There is a shower in each sauna room, as well as a cold water faucet for filling handy galvanized buckets. The idea is to take a cooler by pouring cold water over your head, or asking a friend to throw a bucket on your back. Delicious.

There are private dressing rooms adjoining each sauna room and tub room. The small, clean rooms have a rug on the floor, a bench along one side, electric outlet, mirror and a stack of towels and soft white sheets for wrapping around yourself; paper slippers are also provided. You may take as long as you like in the dressing room after your sauna. And here is where you will want your basic bag, described on the preceding pages.

The hot tubs here are spectacular, beautifully set in their spaces with hanging plants, glowing redwood sides, decks and benches. There is one good-sized redwood tub in a cozy room, white walled and skylighted. Two private dressing rooms, entered from the hall, open into the tub room. There is a shower in the tub room, and the temperature generally hovers around 90 degrees. There is no clock or timer in this room, but the staff will call out 30-minute time, when you are expected to return to your dressing room so that the next customer can enter the tub from the adjacent dressing room.

A giant new hot tub has just been installed which is open to the sun and stars overhead. By removing the ceiling of a large room, the management has created a lovely courtyard, peaceful and serene, a delight to eye and senses.

Massage at Albany Sauna is by arrangement, and lasts the standard half-hour or hour. It is generally an Esalen-type, light massage. If you have arranged for a massage following your sauna, the masseuse will knock on the door of the dressing room at the appointed time and lead you to the massage room. Towels and sheets are provided for you to wrap in; carry your basic bag and clothes to the massage room where you will dress before leaving.

A juice and tea bar is adjacent to the massage rooms. The fruit juices are in a large refrigerator—serve yourself and pay at the counter; the tea shop is also self-service. There are healthy snack foods available and pleasant wooden tables facing the street. We found ourselves sinking gratefully onto benches, dreamily sipping tea until our limp legs could carry us out to the street.

ALBANY SAUNA, 1002 Solano Avenue, Albany, California 94706. Telephone: (415) 525-6262. No overnight accommodations. Tea room with drinks and nutritious snacks. By reservation or drop in. Children welcome. No pets. Cards: BA, MC, VISA. Open daily, noon to 10:30.
Spa facilities: hot tubs, $3.50; sauna, $3; massage, $10 for one-half hour, $18 for one hour and sauna; group and children's rates available. Skin care products sold at desk. Bathing suits optional.

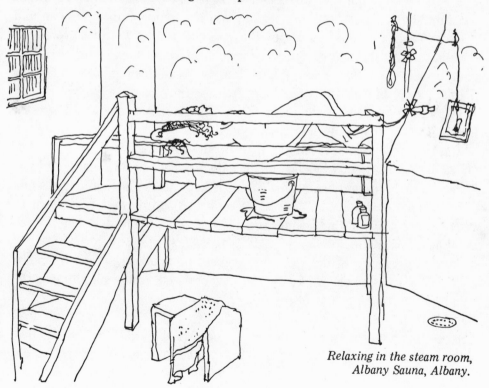

Relaxing in the steam room,
Albany Sauna, Albany.

AMERICAN FAMILY SAUNA & TUB
Richmond and Oakland

A spic and span sauna and tub within a stone's throw of Richmond's Civic Center, American Family is housed in the rear of a small home similar to others on this side street just off busy MacDonald Avenue. This converted residential facility has been in Richmond for many years, although recently taken over by new, young owners who have just opened a branch in Oakland. The Richmond sauna thus has a built-in clientele of "regulars," whereas the Oakland facility is a delightful surprise to North Berkeley/Oakland residents who have been enjoying the recent development of the College Avenue area.

Richmond

The senior member of the American Family has two saunas and two outdoor hot tubs. Each sauna holds six persons and the temperature hovers around 170 degrees. A unique feature of these saunas is that you can lower the temperature by sprinkling water on the rocks without moving an inch from your bench; a simple tug on a pulley line overhead does not let you off at the next stop, but, in Rube Goldberg fashion, opens a valve that releases an even spray of water over the rocks. Each sauna opens to two small dressing rooms. Towels, soap and robes are provided.

The tubs, one smaller (accommodating four) and one larger (accommodating eight) are made of fiberglass set in redwood decking. Both are outdoors in fenced-in back-yard enclosures. Water is kept at 105 to 106 degrees and the tubs are equipped with Jacuzzi jet sprays. A shower area is adjacent to the tub, and you will find a timer and a buzzer to the front desk here as well as in the sauna rooms.

American Family Sauna gives you a pleasant hour away from home or office in a sparkly clean and homey atmosphere—you walk through the laundry room to get to one of the tubs.

College Avenue

The College Avenue shop had just opened at the time we visited. The cheerful front lobby has a beautiful hand-crafted checker set at a small table for two, in addition to oatmeal-colored, contemporary couches.

Three saunas, each done in cedar, open onto private dressing rooms in typical sauna design. Atypical is the arrangement of one of the three saunas; it opens to a large dressing room and a hot tub room, so that a group of 12 may share the area as long as six are "tubbers" and six prefer sauna. (While one can shift from tub to sauna, it is advisable to do one or the other.)

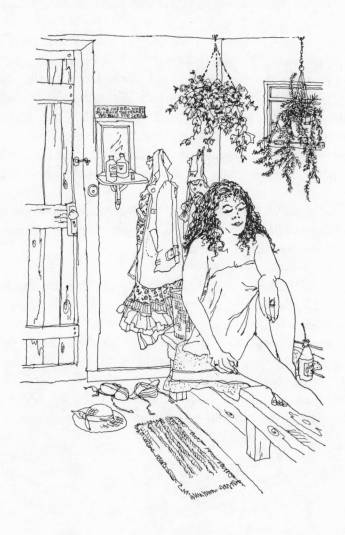

Two other hot tubs are available, each opening to two private dressing rooms that can be used simultaneously by a group or alternated—when you leave the tub room, you buzz the desk from your dressing room so that those in the adjacent room can enter the tub room. Showers, of course, are in the tub room and a dispenser of peppermint soap and a scrub brush is there for your use. (Sauna rooms contain a dispenser of almond liquid soap.)

As in the Richmond facility, tubs are fiberglass set in redwood, but unlike Richmond, all tubs are indoors. Unique to the tubs in this shop is a wonderful "bubbler" action in addition to the familiar jet sprays. Two buttons on the wall allow you to select bubbler or jet, or to alternate. Unlike the jet sprays which come out from the side of the tub, the bubblers leap up vertically from openings in the bench within the tub. When you sit right in the bubbler spray, the water massages your entire torso. Both the jet sprays and bubbler action are on one side of the tub only so that one person can sit right in it while another soaks on the opposite side where the water is quieter.

Only the College Avenue shop offers massage, and appointments must be made in advance. College Avenue intends to put in a line of organic beauty aids, probably the Swedish Glöda products.

AMERICAN FAMILY SAUNA AND TUB, 242 25th Street, Richmond, California 94804. Telephone: (415) 234-1012. 5498 College Avenue, Oakland, California 94618. Telephone: (415) 654-8483. No overnight accommodations. No meal service; mineral water and soft drinks available. Reservations only with credit card or cash deposit. Cards: BA, MC, VISA. Open 12 to 10; closed Monday.

Spa facilities: sauna, $2.75 to $3.50; hot tubs, $3 to $3.50; massage, $15 for 45 minutes, by advance appointment only.

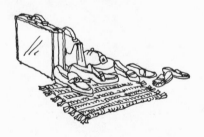

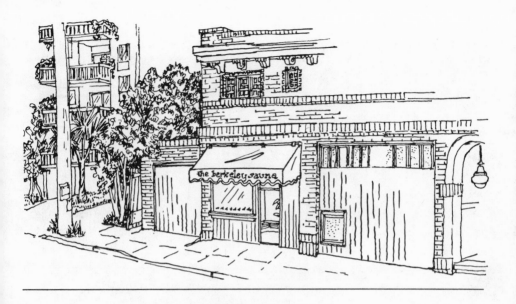

BERKELEY SAUNA
Berkeley

Serene and classy, this small gem of a spa knows exactly what it is about: offering exclusively Swedish saunas in fragrant, spacious rooms in a serene, efficient atmosphere. Located in the center of Berkeley off University Avenue, Berkeley Sauna is straightforward in its service and beautifully appointed. The tasteful redwood store front has the establishment name in gold letters on the plate-glass window through which the afternoon sun streams into a finely proportioned waiting room. The light glints off spotless white plaster walls and reflects softly on the red tile floors. Carpeted stairways take you to a loft hall that leads to the saunas and dressing rooms. Staff and owners work quickly and efficiently from a desk area in the waiting room.

Reservations are honored on time, and you are promptly ushered to your redwood dressing room. All the rooms are remarkably soundproof, further enhancing the peaceful mood of the place.

The saunas occupy four spacious rooms with adjacent private dressing rooms, arranged along a central hall, and contain seats and benches for

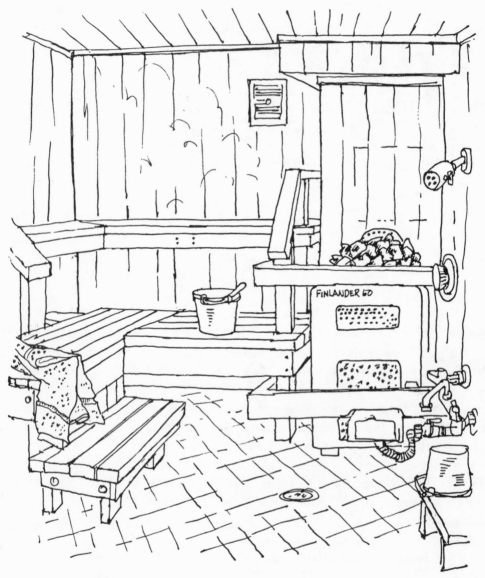

Berkeley Sauna room.

74

sitting and lying. The temperature is controlled at approximately 155 degrees. As in all classic Swedish saunas, there are open charcoal stoves with water bucket and ladle nearby so that you can pour water on the coals for steam. The sauna rooms also contain standing showers and low foot showers, from which you can fill buckets of water to cool yourself. The heady scent of redwood permeates the rooms.

The management suggests that you stay in their saunas for only 10 minutes, retiring at that time for a rest in your dressing room, then a return to the sauna for another 10 minutes. Clear instructions are printed on neat wall signs. The signs further caution: "If at any time you feel uncomfortable in the sauna, return to the dressing room to rest. Sauna floors are slippery when wet. People with medical problems should consult their physician before using the sauna."

Massage is available by appointment only. You should specify masseur or masseuse and whether you wish an hour or half-hour massage. The staff changes from time to time, and on our visit we were given a thorough, excellent deep-muscle massage; inquire as to the style of massage available when you make an appointment.

Towels, soap, bath brush and hair dryer are provided, so come as you are. Juice or mineral water may be purchased at the desk and taken with you to the dressing room.

BERKELEY SAUNA, 1947 Milvia, Berkeley, California 94704. Telephone: (415) 845-8595. No overnight accommodations. Reservations recommended. Children welcome. No pets. Cards: BA, MC. Open daily except Tuesday, noon to 10.
Spa facilities: sauna, $3.50; shower, massage; children's rates available. Juice and skin care products sold at desk. Bathing suits optional.

TASSAJARA HOT SPRINGS
Monterey County

Tassajara Hot Springs is a total experience, allowing you access to beautiful hot springs in a flowing creek bed near accommodations unique in California. Tassajara Hot Springs is part of the Zen Mountain Center, a retreat run by Zen monks and students who live here year round. The Tassajara center is affiliated with the San Francisco and Green Gulch Zen Centers of Northern California.

Tassajara is reached by driving to Carmel Valley Village, then proceding southeast on Carmel Valley Road (G 16) to Jamesburg, a small town where Tassajara maintains offices. Here you may leave your car and continue in four-wheel-drive transportation provided by the Zen Center. If you choose to drive in, you will continue over the 14-mile, dirt Tassajara Road. Your destination is in a canyon of the coastal mountain range that rises up from the spectacular coastline of Monterey County. Press on through the dust. In winter this road is usually impassable due to mud and mud slides, but in the months of May to September, the drive is spectacular.

As early as 1890 there is written record of Tassajara Hot Springs at the head of Arroyo Seco in Monterey County. These hot and sulfurous waters, admittedly difficult to reach by foot or horseback, were considered a tonic by early settlers. One note we ran across in a book by Dr. Winslow Anderson entitled *Mineral Springs and Health Resorts of California* (1890): "Spanish and aborigines in the vicinity frequented these springs for many years and were apparently much benefited."

The atmosphere at Tassajara is calm and serene for the visitor; even the industry of the students is measured and peaceful.

The routine at Tassajara may be one of your own choosing, but we strongly recommend that for at least one day of your stay you participate in the routine of the Zen students. You are most welcome to join part or all of the daily activities at Tassajara. The morning gong rouses students for meditation at four o'clock. You may sit in meditation with the students in the Zendo (the main meeting and meditation house at Tassajara), help in the

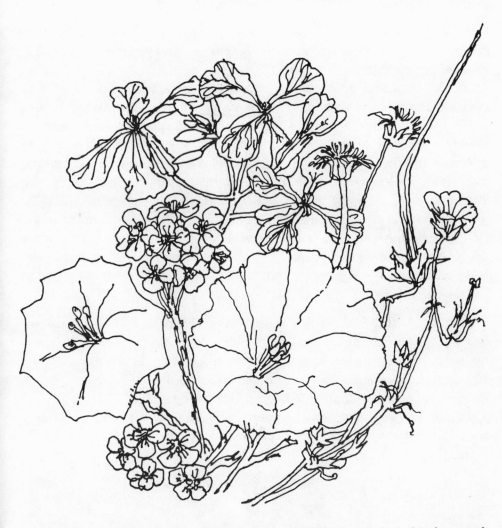

assigned work for the day in gardens or around the grounds or kitchen, and proceed through the day with meals and further meditation. Keep in mind that this vigorous routine is the modified or summer schedule.

Tassajara baths offer a complete range of natural water experience from a dip in the creek to laps in the cold-water swimming pool. The natural waters here are trapped and held at a variety of temperatures. There is a large pool house beside the creek into which the hot spring water flows. Temper the heat with cold water from the creek mixed in individual tubs in the large bath building. Men's and women's bathing is separate in the bathhouses and further down the creek, where it broadens and deepens into a pool big enough for swimming.

Should you stay only for the day and use the baths, you will need to bring your own food. Guests who stay overnight eat with the students and monks in the dining room. The food is the most delicious that the community of Tassajara and the good earth can concoct. Most vegetables and fruits are grown in the fields you see around you. The good food here has become internationally known through the popularity of their recipe books, *The Tassajara Cookbook* and *The Tassajara Bread Book.* Vegetarian, naturally.

Accommodations are sparse and rustic. The most elegant room is the stone room, the only one with a private bath. The redwood cabins with double beds can sleep two people. You share a bath with the adjoining cabin. Bring all personal articles with you to Tassajara; they furnish soap, towels and linens.

TASSAJARA HOT SPRINGS, Carmel Valley, California 93924. Telephone: (408) 659-2229. Accommodations: stone room with private bath, redwood cabins with shared baths; double beds; no telephones; no television. Rates: $26 to $32, three meals included. Reservations required. Children welcome. No pets. No credit cards accepted. Open May to September.
Spa facilities: hot tubs, mineral-water swimming pool, natural rock-lined pools, natural creek pool; $4 for day use; no charge for overnight guests. Bathing suits optional. Separate men's and women's bathing.

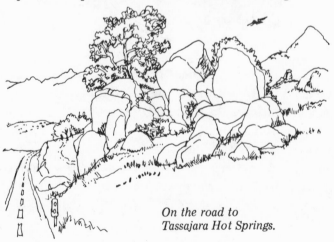

*On the road to
Tassajara Hot Springs.*

ESALEN HOT SPRINGS
Big Sur, Monterey County

Esalen, 300 miles north of Los Angeles and 175 miles south of San Francisco, cliff-hangs dramatically above the shoreline of the fabled Monterey Coast with the Santa Lucia Range rising closely behind. The property has natural hot springs, formed into baths, and was once the home of an Indian tribe known as Esalen. After you leave Monterey, driving down Highway 1 from San Francisco, look for Nepenthe which is 11 miles north of Esalen. A lighted sign on the ocean side of the highway reads: Esalen Institute—By Reservation Only.

Esalen is renowned worldwide, not only as the home of the human potential movement, but also as a place of stunning beauty set on the edge of the Pacific Ocean. It nestles, surrounded by its emerald green lawns and Monterey cyprus groves, snug as a bird's aerie against the dramatic cliffs of the Big Sur coastline.

The hot tubs are dug from the cliffs which fall precipitously to the ocean's edge. The handsome redwood and concrete structure housing the baths projects out from the cliff edge, so that as one sits in the baths, the view of sky and ocean is unimaginably vast and breathtaking. This is easily the most beautiful setting of hot tubs in the world. In addition to the baths, a large outdoor heated swimming pool is located on the grounds.

Esalen itself, the grounds and lodgings, are peaceful, much like a small, quiet resort. People in residence are all taking courses or seminars, attending to the housekeeping and maintenance of Esalen, or permanent members of the faculty in residence.

Essentially Esalen is a center for experimental education in the behavioral sciences, religion and philosophy; the hot baths are just an added bonus. The main business is workshops and seminars that anyone may attend. But the hot baths as well as the grounds of Esalen are accessible only to students enrolled in these workshops. Rooms are always shared by two or three people, usually participants in the same workshop.

Meals at Esalen are an experience unto themselves. You could feast on the view alone. In the dining room the low ceiling and intimate grouping of tables centered with flowers and candles give a feeling of relaxed graciousness. Then you raise your eyes from this inviting scene to a sweep of green lawn dropping abruptly to the crashing Pacific and the limitless blue sky. The dining room is surrounded by a terrace for those who prefer to eat in the full sun or under a shaded eave. Much of the delicious, fresh food prepared at Esalen is grown on the grounds. Thick soups, crisp salads and freshly baked bread were our favorites. Begin a perfect day at Esalen with yourself and breakfast: honey and tea, thick slices of fresh buttered wheat bread, poached eggs; the privacy of a terrace corner in the gentle morning sun enjoying the sound of the ocean, birds pecking the crumbs at your feet; and the promise of a morning in the hot steamy baths alternating with massage and sleep.

And of course, Esalen is famous for its massage. Massage weekends are given frequently and typically center around the baths. A weekend massage workshop for beginners, taught by the Esalen massage crew, usually begins with dinner on Friday night, followed by an introductory talk and an outline of the plan for the weekend. The members of the massage crew give instruction and help the group to practice basic techniques of massage upon one another. Sensory awareness is stressed: "As we learn to feel with our hands how the body and the life-force within it works, we learn to release tensions in others and to be more fully aware of ourselves."

There is an excellent book store on the grounds, stocked with a selection of titles on the human potential movement, including books on massage and hot springs. Lotions and potions may also be purchased here.

We advise bringing warm sweaters to Esalen year round; the nights are quite cool. Comfortable, informal, loose clothing and your basic bag will see you through. Do not forget hiking shoes if you are interested in the trails which leave Esalen and branch into the Santa Lucia mountains.

Guests traveling to Esalen by air or bus may be met at the Monterey Airport or the Greyhound Terminal at five o'clock each Sunday and Friday; cost is $15 per person one way. The Esalen office must be notified of your time of arrival in order to insure limousine service.

ESALEN HOT SPRINGS, Esalen Institute, Big Sur, California 93920. Telephone: (408) 667-2335 or (213) 820-5511. Accommodations: double occupancy rooms; shared bath; double and single beds; no telephones; no television. Rates: from $60 per person for a weekend to over $1500 for a month-long workshop, tuition, food, lodging and use of all facilities included. Reservations required. Children not allowed. No pets. Cards: AE, BA, MC. Open all year.

Spa facilities: hot mineral baths, massage, included in seminar fee. Bathing suits optional in hot baths.

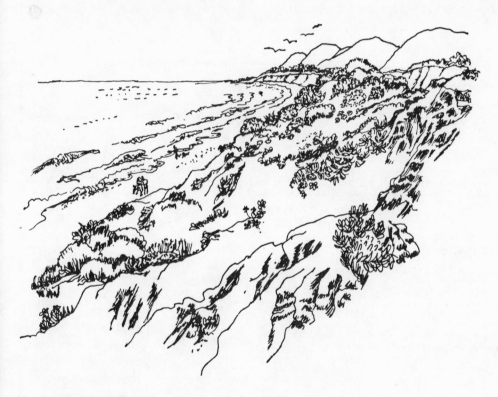

Northern California beach.

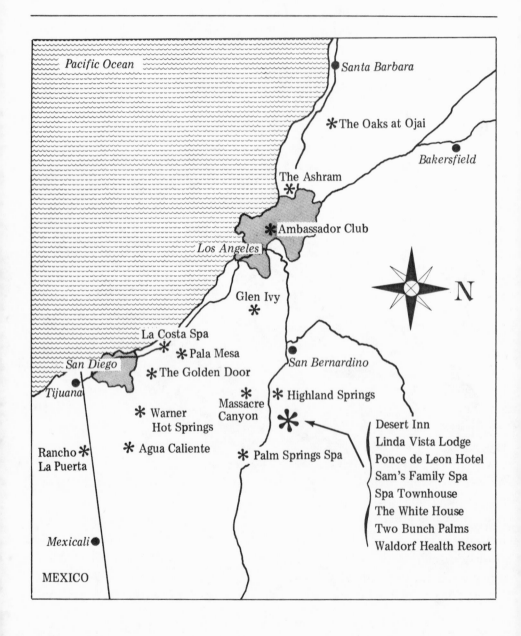

Pacific Ocean

● Santa Barbara

✳ The Oaks at Ojai

● Bakersfield

The Ashram
✳

✳ Ambassador Club

Los Angeles

Glen Ivy
✳

La Costa Spa
✳ ✳ Pala Mesa
✳ The Golden Door

San Diego

Tijuana

● San Bernardino

✳ Highland Springs

Massacre
Canyon
✳

✳ Warner
Hot Springs

Rancho ✳
La Puerta

✳ Agua Caliente

✳ Palm Springs Spa

✳

→ Desert Inn
Linda Vista Lodge
Ponce de Leon Hotel
Sam's Family Spa
Spa Townhouse
The White House
Two Bunch Palms
Waldorf Health Resort

Mexicali ●

MEXICO

N

82

THE OAKS AT OJAI
Ojai, Ventura County

A description of The Oaks at Ojai is a most appropriate introduction to the southern California section of this book. For The Oaks is typical of those large southern California health resorts that have come to characterize the best of American spas. The Oaks, Rancho la Puerta, The Golden Door, The Ashram, La Costa have in common excellent staffs and programs devoted to physical fitness and relaxation.

These programs are conducted over several days or weeks in a live-in arrangement. You check in and devote yourself totally to a regime of good, low-calorie nutrition, as much exercise as you can stand, alternating with periods of rest and relaxation, followed by massage and hot-water soaks, and a deep night's sleep. When you leave a week or more later, you are pounds lighter, in exhilarating physical shape, deeply rested, and committed to a continuing program of self-fitness.

All these large California health spas have highly professional, well-integrated regimes of exercise, nutrition and sport. They are adept at applying the latest, most effective modes of fitness training and supervision to your particular body. Don't be surprised if annual return visits become a part of your life.

On entering the Oaks a quick look around will give the alert observer an immediate sense of the key characteristic of this spa—people hurry by, smiling, talking among themselves, wearing every form of sport attire. The mood is buoyant, highly energetic and most congenial. The Oaks is surely the happiest of the spas we visited.

Guests at The Oaks, like guests at all the large southern California health resorts, come from around the United States and the globe. A man from Denmark said, "Where else can you spend 40 dollars a day and feel like a million? I spend at least two weeks at this place every year. Staying healthy." One woman we talked with was getting in shape for a two-month work tour of the Far East. "I exercise hard in the morning, walk three miles a day, read and talk all afternoon, soak in hot water whenever I feel like it . . . and leave here with enough energy for months of work." A couple on

Vegetable stand near Ojai.

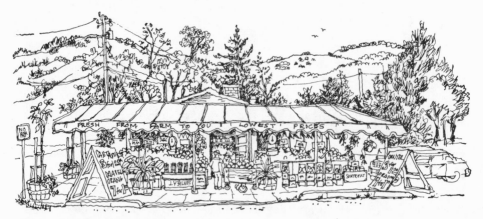

the early morning walk came to the Oaks to lose weight and improve their tennis. A lady from New York remarked at dinner, "Listen, it's different out here. I leave all that work and noise in New York. For me this is a retreat. This is where I come to recharge."

The Oaks at Ojai is relatively new, and just coming into its own in accommodations and popularity. It is located 90 miles from Los Angeles on Highway 33; the drive there is a scenic delight, whether you are coming from Highway 5 or Highway 101. The climate is warm during the day and cool at night, perfect resort weather.

The Oaks offers the wide range of spa activities for men and women common to large California health resorts; their water exercise and general fitness programs are outstanding.

Sheila Cluff is the owner and manager of The Oaks at Ojai and The Palms at Palm Springs, a new fitness resort scheduled to open in early 1979. She is also president of Physical Fitness Inc., a company that has developed and teaches physical fitness programs in this country and abroad. She is assisted in the exercise program by Karma Kientzler, and both women, with care and intelligence, will carefully work out a fitness plan for you, individually.

A typical day's workout may include a brisk walk or jog beginning at seven. Although you may choose to begin your day anytime, if you want the full benefit of a week at The Oaks, you'll start early. After breakfast, stretch classes begin in the exercise room, followed by a faster paced class for a more vigorous muscle work-out and cardiovascular benefits.

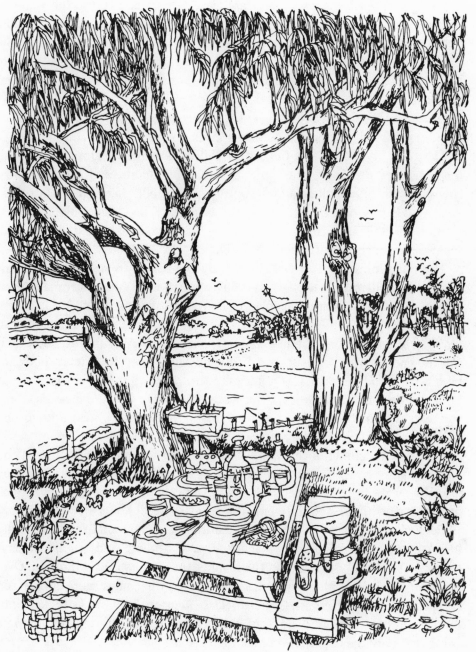

Lake near Ojai.

Pool exercises begin at 11 and are cleverly designed to use the water as resistance for body contouring and self-massage. The water is a comfortable temperature, the sky clear and sparkling blue, the company lively, the exercises wonderfully invigorating. We noticed everyone piling into the pool at 11, and then again at two for another hour's session, with Sheila and Karma as Pied Pipers.

Other periods in the day are spent at tennis, playing golf, in yoga or dance class, or just resting around the pool or in the lounges.

The food at The Oaks is limited to 750 well-balanced calories a day. All the meals are delicious, the fresh vegetables and fruits, and natural, whole foods beautifully cooked and tastefully presented; there are no artificial additives. If you do not intend to lose weight at The Oaks, a higher-calorie menu will be planned for you. Special menus are also planned under medical supervision for those with medical problems.

The nutritionist at The Oaks will teach you how to prepare menus for your special dietary needs when you return home. Recipes for all foods prepared at The Oaks are available in a convenient packet of individual cards.

The Oaks has good massage technicians and they recommend a most sensible series of steps before and after massage. A sauna or hot tub is recommended prior to massage to unwind and loosen up a tense body, or even a tired body. Take a few minutes to turn your attention inward to your body. During massage, close your eyes and talk very little. Massage is a time for relaxation, refreshment. Take a fantasy journey in your mind to any place you enjoy, such as the ocean or the forest.

Feel free to communicate with your massage technician about the firmness or lightness of the touch. Many people enjoy a massage most when they are stiff and sore from rigorous exercise, and others love the deep relaxation just before bedtime. Appointments can be made at all hours at The Oaks.

Generally, massage heightens circulation of the blood, so it naturally increases the flow of blood to all parts of the body, and the benefits of massage are usually seen first in the blanket that covers us all—the skin. Over a period of time, with regular massage, the skin becomes more supple and radiant. Deep muscle massage may release tensions and stress locked into muscle contractions. And none of this verbage touches the feeling of well-being that only the experience of a good massage can evoke.

Dress is as informal as the atmosphere at The Oaks. Be sure to bring along sports gear for tennis, horseback riding, golf or fishing, walking or running—and a warm sweater and jacket for evening strolls in the town or surrounding countryside.

THE OAKS AT OJAI, 122 East Ojai Avenue, Ojai, California 93023. Telephone: (805) 646-5573 or (213) 550-8075. Accommodations: air-conditioned rooms in shaded bungalows around pool or guest rooms with balcony in the main lodge; private baths; telephones; television. Rates: from $39 per person, per day triple occupancy to $63 per person, per day single occupancy; three meals daily, snacks and beverages, medical supervision, fitness classes and complete use of resort facilities included. By reservation only. Children not permitted. No pets. Cards: AE, BA, MC, VISA. Open all year. *Spa facilities:* physical fitness program, hot tubs with Jacuzzi, swimming pool, sauna, massage, beauty care, yoga and dance classes, golf, tennis, horseback riding.

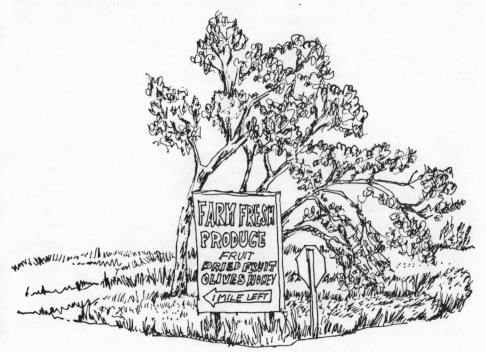

THE ASHRAM
Calabasas, Los Angeles County

In a California-modern stucco house 30 minutes west of Los Angeles and just inland from the Pacific Ocean, a few people who are dedicated to being superfit work their way through the most vigorous program available for amateurs in California. Although Olympic team members and professional athletes do train here from time to time, most of the runners bounding along these hilly trails are simply getting in shape to live their lives in top physical form.

The Ashram is unique among spas in this book, for while it is a retreat with natural waters, pools, gym and health regimen, it is not a place to go for rest and relaxation. Instead it presents the maximum challenge that your body can tolerate in a fast-paced, seven-day regime of muscle building, cardiovascular training, fasting and meditation. The Ashram is for people who are willing to practice the difficult and often painful daily disciplines that lead to the rewarding exhiliration of peak physical shape. There is a sincere attempt here at integrating activities for mind, body and spirit in the daily routine and the program is more successful than most in tailoring diet and exercise to individual needs. That is precisely why they accept only six to eight people at a time.

Your stay at the Ashram begins in the same spirit that guides the week—simple, austere, concentrated. You arrive without car (there are pick-ups at or near the airport) bringing only running shoes, socks, bathing suit and toothbrush. Other clothing—sweatshirt, T-shirt, robe and kaftan—are furnished and neatly folded on the twin bed in your double room.

Upon your arrival you will be given a medical check-up by Dr. Anne-Marie Bennstrom who created the spa, or by energetic and enlivening Dr. Catharina Hedberg who manages the programs. At this time a personal record is begun of your stay at the spa, diet and fasting are discussed with you, and your "biological age " based upon your state of physical fitness is computed. Most people are amazed to find that at age 30, they have a biological age of 56.

Basically the food at the Ashram is juice and tea and vitamins with some raw vegetables and melons. Meals are taken communally around a large table opening onto the patio. The Ashram is an intimate experience in group living as well as a tough training camp.

The day begins at six o'clock with morning yoga and meditation in a beautiful wood and glass dome perched atop a hill overlooking the rolling coastal hills around Los Angeles. After a breakfast of juice and bran the two- to four-mile morning hike begins. This long hike is repeated in the evening in the hills or on the beach. The pace is fast and the trails lead up steep hills and down sharp inclines. The air is clear and cool; the trail passes through natural gardens of wild lilac and buckweed, sumac and sage.

The bulk of the day is spent in hour-long exercise classes, in lifting weights, or in water with more exercise or fast games of water volleyball. The jogging track circles around a beautiful wooded glade with a wide creek of cool, swift-flowing water. In the shadiest area, the creek has been widened to make a deep pool some 20 yards in diameter. After a hot run you plunge in here to cool, float and stretch out your aching limbs. The main exercise pool is heated and the warm water is delicious to tired muscles. Massage is superb.

Meditation and yoga were led by Catharina during our stay at The Ashram. She states firmly: "The physical fitness must be your foundation to greater self-awareness and it comes first. After that each person is given the opportunity for relaxation, for mental growth and awareness through meditation. We want each person to retain the growth of their week here—meditation practice, change in diet, elimination of coffee and cigarettes. I also see the Ashram as a growing ground for our staff. This is a growth experience for us all."

THE ASHRAM, P.O. Box 8, Calabasas, California 91302. Telephone: (213) 888-0232. Accommodations: double rooms in large house; no telephones or television. Rates: $800 per week, Sunday to Saturday, meals and complete program included. Deposit of $300 required within 10 days of making reservation. Children under 18 not permitted. No pets. No credit cards.
Spa facilities: exercise pool, gymnasium, massage, yoga.

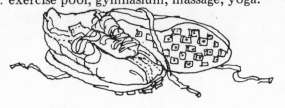

AMBASSADOR TENNIS & HEALTH CLUB
Los Angeles

The inclusion of the Ambassador Tennis and Health Club in a book whose focus is hot waters requires some explanation. Most spas located in southern California cities are gymnasiums, which may include saunas or Jacuzzi tubs filled with heated city water. These health centers, devoted to body-building, weight loss and fitness, if properly described, would fill a second volume. So we have restricted our review to a large, accessible, typical urban spa of southern California, The Ambassador Tennis and Health Club. The selection is particularly appropriate as accommodations are available at the Ambassador Hotel, although many of the rooms have not been modernized. A stay here, combined with a daily work-out at the Tennis and Health Club, makes a model urban spa experience.

Los Angeles' newest and most complete tennis club and health spa is located on the grounds of the venerable Ambassador Hotel on busy Wilshire Boulevard. This vintage hotel has always been a country resort in the middle of town, surrounded by acres of grounds, cottages, plush restaurants and lounges. Its history, replete with razzmatazz, stretches back to the earliest days of Hollywood and movie-industry growth.

Ground was broken for the Ambassador in 1919, and when the hotel opened to guests in 1921, the press acclaimed it one of the most stimulating and plush hotels in the world. There was no Wilshire Boulevard at the time, just a dirt road and miles of open country. From the beginning, though, Angelenos embraced the hotel as their home-town community hall. The Academy Awards presentations have been held here numerous times, as well as gala Hollywood parties, weddings, proms, bar mitzvahs, and movie premières. Checking in at the Ambassador, you walk through the same door that has opened for Will Rogers and Harry Belafonte, for queens, kings and emperors from around the world.

The Tennis and Health Club is located on the grounds behind the main hotel buildings and adjacent to the big swimming pool where bodies beautiful still tan while sipping and sighing and waiting for the Big Discovery. Most of the guests, however, are swimming laps, or resting between fast games on the court or a workout in the newly refurbished gym.

The membership in the Tennis and Health Club is coed, approximately 40 percent women and 60 percent men. The sexes have separate locker and sauna rooms, but all other facilities and classes are shared.

Sauna, whirlpool baths and the Olympic-size swimming pool comprise the heat and water therapies available. Gym and exercise rooms are spacious, carpeted, mirrored, and open onto the fresh air and sun of the pool area. Competent yoga instructors, members of the Yoga Association of Southern California, give classes on a regular daily schedule; these classes are free to members. Massage is available by arrangement and reservation at the club desk. The jogging track is small. A raised track in the middle of the hotel gardens, it will suffice for a warmup, but not for a workout. Tennis is the major attraction at this spa. The club has 10 new outdoor tennis courts, with night lights and pros in residence for teaching individuals or classes.

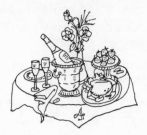

AMBASSADOR TENNIS AND HEALTH CLUB, 3400 Wilshire Boulevard, Los Angeles, California 90010. Telephone: (213) 385-6487. Accommodations: hotel rooms, garden bungalows, luxury suites; private baths; telephones; television. Rates: $34 to $46 single, $42 to $54 double, hotel rooms; $38 to $50 single, $48 to $60 double, bungalows; suites from $70. Three restaurants in hotel. Reservations advised. Children welcome. No pets. Cards: AE, BA, CB, DC, MC, VISA. Open all year.
Spa facilities: sauna, whirlpool, exercise room, yoga, gym equipment, Olympic-size swimming pool, putting green, jogging track. Rates: swimming pool, putting green and jogging track, no charge for hotel guests; $7.50 per day for use of other facilities by hotel guests; $500 initiation fee, plus yearly or monthly membership fees for non-registered guests.

GLEN IVY HOT SPRINGS
Corona, Riverside County

Vic and Carol Summers recently bought the old Glen Ivy Hot Springs Resort and are pouring in a tremendous amount of young energy and skill to bring the spa back to its earlier beauty—before it was damaged by repeated fires and allowed to deteriorate.

At the base of the Cleveland National Forest mountain range, Glen Ivy is situated in one of the most beautiful natural settings in the state. Although the deer have shied back a bit with all of the activity at the resort, they continue to roam the hills behind the spa, while quail, coyote and rabbits still abound in this area, once described as a "sportsman's paradise."

Vic Summers is the self-taught historian for the area and will charm you with the rich history of the resort and colorful anecdotes from its past, as you sit at a poolside table with hawks, orioles and hummingbirds performing all around you. Vic is alert to the fact that a whole new population of "into health" people are discovering the marvel of hot springs, mud bathing and mineral-water soaking. When he took over the resort, the clientele was essentially older Europeans seeking relief from arthritic pain, but he anticipates an influx of younger people in the near future.

Hard at work giving the entire facility a "face lift," Vic has placed redwood siding over the concrete-block exterior of the old bathhouse. He has also opened the truly lovely Cafe Glen Ivy with red quarry-tile tables and photographs on the walls showing the evolution of the spa from the 1800s. The cafe serves sandwiches, salads, fruits and juices—all elegantly fresh and eye-appealing. Much outside planting has been done in the past few years. From poolside, it is a real "eye trip" to look out at the succulents, verbena and oleander. Especially striking is the bougainvillea climbing its way up a massive tree trunk.

Open for day use only, Glen Ivy has two large pools, one a mineral-water swimming pool maintained at approximately 90 degrees and the other a hotter therapy pool which is far bigger than most of the hot therapy pools we have seen. Facing the pools is a row of individual tiled tubs—the whirlpool baths—where water normally comes in at 106 degrees; these tubs are equipped with guard rails on each side. Behind the pools is a beautiful shaded picnic area, flanked by a large sulphur mud bath, also lightly shaded and semi-secluded. Each tub has guard rails on the sides and stairs within the tub so that one immerses oneself in the hot water literally by steps.

The massage/sauna building located behind the pool area also has undergone considerable work. According to the Summers, time and neglect had perhaps taken their worst toll on this building. When you enter the building, you are faced with a reception counter—the Lotions and Potions shop developed by Carol Summers to sell the organic skin care products she imports from Arizona. Men's and women's quarters have separate entryways, rest rooms and dressing rooms, but they share the same spa facilities, although at different times. These include two massage rooms, two large redwood saunas that exude the pungent fragrance of eucalyptus oils, and four private hot mineral baths.

An example of the conscientious energy being invested in Glen Ivy's restoration is the massive black lettering outside the locker/dressing rooms. To designate the men's and women's entrances, Vic wanted a bold oversize typeface. He found the type he wanted but it was not available in a size large enough to be dramatic. Being a dabbler in graphics, he took the letters in the size available and rounded up projection equipment to enlarge the images, which he carefully traced to make his own giant letters. He is justly proud of

Mineral water pools, Glen Ivy Hot Springs.

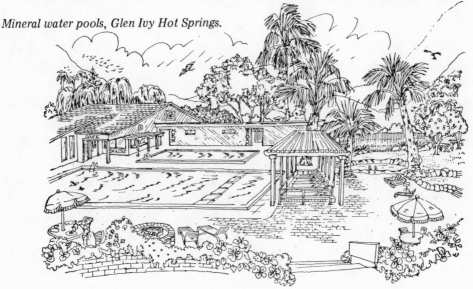

his signs, which probably can be read from the old lodge high on the hill, where he and Carol and their staff now live.

Although Glen Ivy does not have overnight accommodations, the separately owned and operated Glen Ivy Recreational Vehicle Park, at the base of the hill, provides campsites at a nominal charge for spa enthusiasts. The park also offers its own tremendously varied facilities—tennis, swimming, games, horseback riding, hiking, recreation hall and "Ivy Pub" for dining and dancing. While an RV park is entirely different in atmosphere from a mineral-water resort and spa, staying here offers a chance to indulge yourself in two contrasting vacation experiences.

For dining in the area in addition to the Cafe Glen Ivy up at the spa and the Ivy Pub at the RV park, there is an incredible place called Tom's Foods whose interior looks like a turn-of-the-century dining room with soft, polished oak tables; the view, however, is of contemporary country landscape, picnic tables and horseback riders. Next to Tom's Foods is Tom's Produce Market. How many times have you passed a country market while driving from here to there and passed it up "for next time"? Here, it is at your fingertips.

The attraction of this resort area is its natural beauty (do bring binoculars and hiking boots), the diversity of activities available, and the affordable price for the whole package.

GLEN IVY HOT SPRINGS, 25000 Glen Ivy Road, Corona, California 91720. Telephone: (714) 737-4723. No overnight accommodations. Cafe. Children welcome. No credit cards accepted. Open Tuesday through Sunday, 10 to 6.
Spa facilities: mineral-water swimming pool, hot therapy pool, individual whirlpool tubs, sulphur mud bath, sauna, $3 for day use. Massage, $7 for 20 minutes, $15 for 45 minutes.

GLEN IVY RECREATIONAL VEHICLE PARK, 24601 Glen Ivy Road, Route 2, Box 95, Corona, California 91720. Telephone: (714) 737-4261. Accommodations: hook-up, $8; space, $7; weekly and monthly rates; higher rates on holiday weekends. "Ivy Pub" dining room. Reservations accepted with full payment in advance. Children welcome. Pets permitted on leash. Cards: BA, MC, VISA. Open all year.

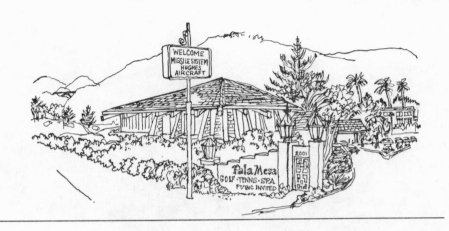

PALA MESA RESORT
Fallbrook, San Diego County

Fallbrook is known for its acres of flower farms, its avocado and orange groves and the very comfortable Pala Mesa Resort, owned and operated by Jim Leonard and his sons. The Leonard family started out to develop one of the best-known golf courses in the state, and having accomplished that, expanded to tennis and then decided to include a health spa.

While the Leonards were wondering where to build a spa on their property, they learned that a nearby 60-acre executive estate, facing lovely Swan Lake, was for sale and they purchased it for their spa.

The resort now offers its guests a choice of two worlds to move in. The lodge, where all guests stay whether or not on the spa program, is a well-appointed motel complex and a sportsman's paradise with its rolling green golf course, pro shop and tennis courts. The spa is a secluded hideaway, festooned with weeping willows and graced with a charming bridge that crosses the lake to a separate structure now used as an exercise room. This choice of environment is perfect for couples who differ on the ideal vacation: One can remain at Pala Mesa's main lodge grounds and play hard all day, stop in the lounge for a cocktail and live a more or less "citified" life. The other can enroll in the spa program.

Actually, there are two spa programs—the weekend "Terrific Toner" and the week-long "Fabulous Conditioner." Arrangements for both are made through the spa director, Bette Spain. The spa accommodates only 10

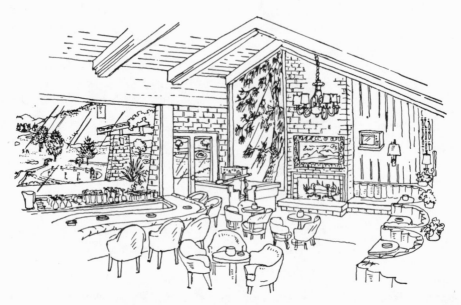

The lounge with view of golf course, Pala Mesa Resort.

persons and is personalized for your needs and wants. It is a co-ed program—men have their own exercise and massage areas—but usually the men opt for the golf and tennis and the women choose the spa.

On a typical visit, you would check into the lodge in the afternoon and saunter over for a cocktail and dinner in the lovely dining room where the green of the carpeting precisely matches the green of the golf course in one enormous indoor-outdoor expanse.

In the morning you join the other spa guests. One of the first names you will hear mentioned with much affection is George. A Czechoslovakian with a wealth of anecdotes and folkloric hints on health, George will probably lead your morning hike around the golf course. You next move to the main lodge for a specially prepared diet breakfast (or a full breakfast if you are not on a weight-reduction program) and then, by van, to the spa property two miles away.

Behind an inviting gateway, you enter a small house with sunken living room and fireplace around which the bedrooms have been converted to massage rooms. A manicure table is off to the side. The living room looks out to Swan Lake and the pool area, where George will lead you through "wake-up" exercises. They are gentle but, if you are out of shape, you will know it. You then walk across a wooden bridge to the exercise room for a 40-minute session of advanced whole-body exercise. These exercises are made very pleasant with music, maracas, poles and comfortable mats and they give your body a head-to-toe stretching and toning. At mid-point a young lady magically appears with a silver tray of stemmed glasses filled with the freshest juice you will ever taste; juices are also available all day from the tiny kitchen in the spa. After a session of guided water exercise in the main pool, a light lunch is served in the spa living room. The afternoon brings more water exercise, followed by leg, thigh and torso toning or spot reducing. In the late afternoon you may schedule a facial, massage, pedicure, manicure, hand/foot reflexology or just loll in the sun.

At five o'clock, the van takes you back to the lodge for an elegant dinner by candlelight.

PALA MESA RESORT, 2001 South Highway 395, Fallbrook, California 92028. Telephone: resort (714) 728-5881, spa (714) 728-6546. Accommodations: rooms in lodge; private baths; double, queen- and king-size beds;

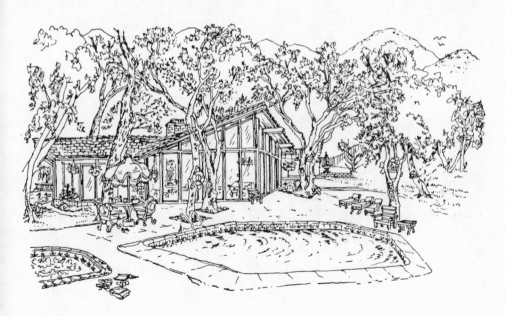

Pools at Pala Mesa.

telephones; color television. Rates: $40 to $48, European plan; group rates for six or more rooms with meals. Dining room with full bar service. Deposit required with reservation. Children welcome. No pets. Cards: BA, MC, VISA. Open all year.

Spa facilities: hikes, Jacuzzi, sauna, aquabics, exercise, facial, massage, scalp massage, hand/foot reflexology, shampoo, set, manicure, pedicure, all meals, special diets and overnight accommodations, $795 per person for one week, $345 per person for weekend; special rates for couples when only one person is on the spa program.

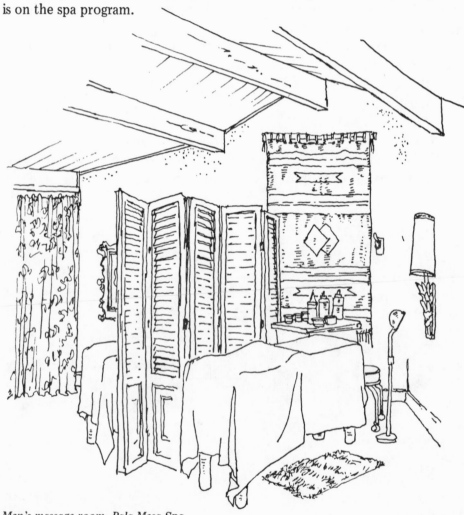

Men's massage room, Pala Mesa Spa.

LA COSTA SPA
Carlsbad, San Diego County

La Costa—the spa of spas—has been given every superlative in a public relations expert's bag of tricks. We agree that everything about La Costa, including the hospitable staff, invites hyperbole.

When you come to the entrance of "Rancho La Costa" after a lovely winding drive around one of Carlsbad's lovely lagoons, you are entering a self-contained village, or small city, where the La Costa Spa is but one of the extensive and elaborate resort features. An aerial view of Rancho La Costa is probably the only way to get an accurate perspective of its scope and splendor.

Here, we shall confine ourselves to a description of the spa, alone, and to the women's section where we enjoyed a "typical" day. The men's quarters, we understand, essentially duplicate the women's facility but provide more extensive gym and work-out programs.

When you first check in at the main reception desk of the spa building, whether on the "spa plan" or using the spa as a hotel guest, you are ushered into your quarters—women in one direction and men in another—and told to "enjoy your day." Your first stop is a semi-circular appointment counter where a staff member sits down with you to plan your day's schedule. The next stop is the locker room where you change into a blue terry wrap-around to which you pin your activities card. The locker room is your "base." Each time you shift activities, you stop back there to change.

La Costa's mineral whirlpool baths, rock steam rooms, saunas, Swiss showers (17 hot/cold sprays), exercise pools, solariums, body conditioning salon, private facial rooms, massage cubicles and beauty salon are wrapped in a wonderland of glass and indoor-outdoor pavilions; you might worry about getting lost but for a cheerful and ever-present staff to lead you through the maze. If you are on a regular spa program, you will be weighed and measured on your first day and at the end of your stay.

Your first stop might be for a facial in a dimly lit, soundproof room where the facialist speaks to you in hushed tones. The room very quickly becomes a sanctuary. After the cleansing and manipulation of your skin and face, she creams your hands and feet and slips them into mittens and booties, plasticized and thermally heated to warm you to toasty comfort. With cool-dipped gauze pads over your eyelids, your body wrapped in a light cotton sheet, and your hands and feet all cuddled in mittens and booties, you will discover that a La Costa facial does, indeed, "make the world go away."

After the facial, you might elect a massage, either in one of the Roman baths or in one of the small interior massage rooms. The Roman baths are perhaps the most striking feature of the spa. These glass-enclosed pavilions open to sun and sky and are surrounded on all sides by corridors where blue-terried ladies move hither and yon. The massage is expertly done in quiet efficiency; be sure to take advantage of the few minutes relaxation time left to you when the masseuse leaves the room rather than leaping up for your next activity. The feast is so sumptuous, there is a temptation to "gulp your food," but the experience should be slowly savored.

Following the massage, you might return to the locker room to change into La Costa's light blue—too soft and lovely to be called a sweat suit—for disco dance in the body-conditioning salon. In front of its wall-to-wall mirror, you may start with a few stretching exercises on your own until the instructor appears. Then bang! The music is on and she is moving to it, barking out dance calls to a straggly chorus line trying to follow the intricate step patterns of disco. It is very easy to get lost and find yourself facing a roomful of blue-suited women when you are supposed to be facing the wall. Some collapse in helpless laughter or simply pick it up again and keep going.

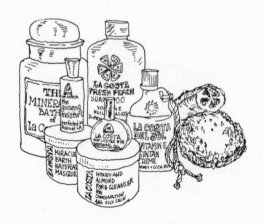

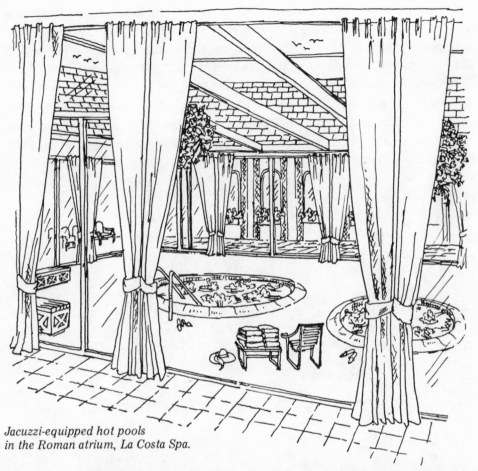

*Jacuzzi-equipped hot pools
in the Roman atrium, La Costa Spa.*

At the end of the 45-minute session, comes a grand finale, complete with walking canes. For a few brief minutes of your life, you can be Liza Minelli.

You might now be ready for yoga exercise. The classes are usually held inside, but on our visit it was conducted on the lawn, which is far nicer for deep breathing and total relaxation. Birds chirp around you, leaves rustle, and the light of the sun filters through the branches to penetrate your closed eyelids.

The rest of the day and week gives you time for a scrub massage with a loufa, an herbal wrap in soft yellow blankets that reflect the glow of the fireplace, and all manner of beauty/body care from the extravaganza of choices offered by La Costa—including daily make-up classes for women.

All guests on the spa plan meet with the dietician and resident physician to go over their objectives for their stay at La Costa—whether they are there to lose, to gain, or to tone. Spa plan guests eat in a special section of the large dining room overlooking the Tournament of Champions golf course. La Costa goes to extraordinary efforts to offer you one of the most well-worked out menus of gourmet low-calorie dishes that you are likely to find. Dieting guests are treated to such delicacies as rock·lobster tails and low-calorie chocolate mousse. Your special menu lists the caloric value of each selection (and gives you ample selections) so that you need make no slips at mealtime. In other words, once your daily caloric intake has been set for you, you

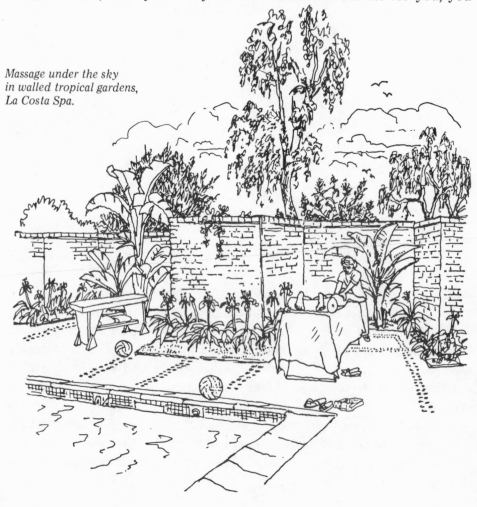

Massage under the sky
in walled tropical gardens,
La Costa Spa.

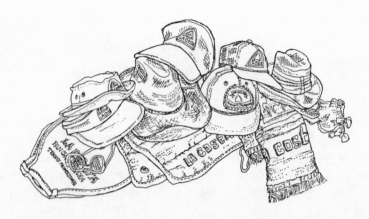

assume responsibility for your dietary program without being tantalized by foods that will sabotage your best intentions.

La Costa offers its hotel guests a remarkable range of leisure activities—practice tennis courts with automatic ball return and closed-circuit video tape to let you see yourself in action, a classic golf course, horseback riding, and much, much more. La Costa's theme is "For people who hate to be bored." If you want the feeling of being totally taken care of, in luxury surroundings, with countless activity choices, La Costa should more than satisfy you.

RANCHO LA COSTA, Carlsbad, California 92008. Telephone: (714) 438-9111. Accommodations: rooms in main building, suites in spa building with patios, studio and one-bedroom cottages with bars; two- and three-bedroom villas with full kitchens and fireplaces, executive homes; private baths; queen-size beds; telephones; color television. Rates: $70 to $140 for rooms only. Four dining rooms. Deposit required with reservation. Children welcome. No pets. Cards: AE, BA, MC. Open all year.

Spa facilities: Spa plan includes accommodations in spa building, diet meals in main dining room, individualized spa program supervised by a physician and dietician, full use of all spa and recreational facilities at La Costa, $150 per day single, $225 per day double, minimum three-night stay. Sauna, steam rooms, Swiss showers, exercise pools, solarium, facials, massage, yoga, disco dance, beauty salon and make-up classes, men's gymnasium and women's body conditioning salon available to Rancho La Costa guests not on spa program at nominal charge.

THE GOLDEN DOOR
Escondido, San Diego County

The Golden Door today stands as the model for small luxury spas through-out the world. Attention to details of service and serenity makes a week at this resort one of the touchstone experiences in anyone's health diary.

Only 33 guests, cared for by a staff of 87 experts with a great love of life and of people, are allowed into this private domain each week. From the moment you pass through the Golden Door (whose surface design is a gem-studded tree of life), you are expected to devote your time and energy to your own life force and to emerge at the end of the week renewed and recharged.

As has been said repeatedly, people do not come to the Golden Door just to lose weight. They come for an overall feeling which can most accurately be called a sense of ease, of well being. As this magic happens, you may also become aware of the great energy and planning which goes into creating this remarkable balance. Not only does the balance come from your own disciplined exercise and deep relaxation, but it is a result of the concern and planning of Deborah Mazzanti, creator of the Golden Door as well as Rancho La Puerta, and her skilled staff.

The Golden Door guards a Japanese-style complex of buildings modeled on the old inns of Japan. It is a beautiful and intimate setting. The plantings and water arrangements in the interior courtyards delight the eye; everywhere are details of architecture and arrangement perfect in design. Indeed, the total, leafy 157 acres of vegetable gardens, walking trails and wooded hillsides have been designed to provide delight for all the senses.

The program of exercises is as rigorous as any we encountered. A typical day might include a sunrise hike, a low-calorie breakfast, stretching exercises, dance therapy, water exercises and massage. After a lunch that rarely exceeds 250 calories, the afternoon is spent in fast physical activity (volleyball in the water, tennis, cardiopulmonary exercises) alternating with periods of total relaxation in steam rooms, herbal wraps, sun baths or meditation.

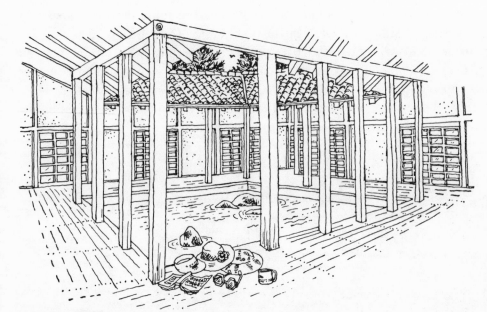

Courtyard, The Golden Door.

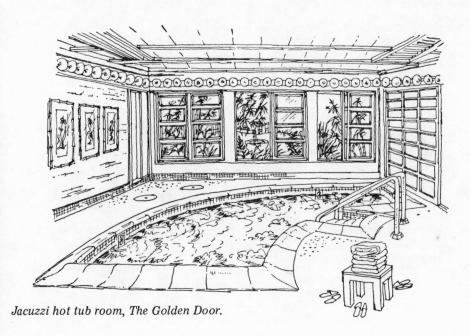

Jacuzzi hot tub room, The Golden Door.

The exercise program is tailored for you by the staff and is designed to be challenging. What you learn in this week at the Golden Door, however, is to divide exercise into small 10 to 30 minute periods with rest in between. "Exercise comes first; rest is the reward." When you return to your busy world, you are advised to spend 10 to 30 minutes on these exercises several times a day to release tension and restore the carbon dioxide/oxygen balance of your body. The result is instant refreshment.

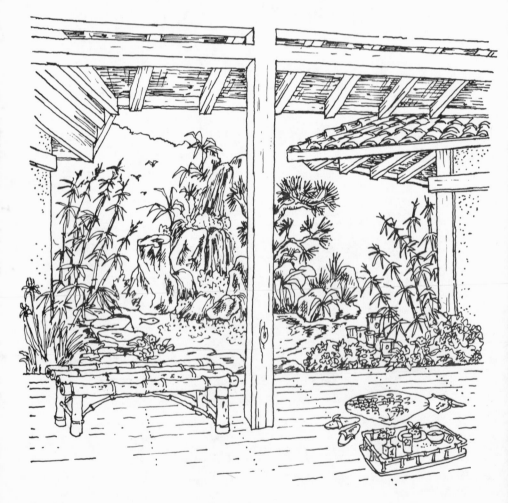

Breakfast in a private garden, The Golden Door.

The bathhouse at Golden Door is a beautiful complex of rooms housing steam room, sauna, showers and Swiss hoses, a fine needle spray of water that the attendant sweeps over your body. There is also a fan-shaped deep warm-water pool where guests congregate in the evening for a family soak. Outdoors are two full-size swimming pools; the water volleyball pool is thoughtfully spread north-to-south so that the sun in your eyes does not interfere with play.

The natural foods at the Golden Door are grown in their own organic gardens. They also raise their own chickens for fresh eggs. The fare is low-calorie, low-sodium, low-cholesterol gourmet. After the first day, we were amazed that our 900-calorie allotment could be so satisfying, and sought out the chef to ask some questions. Spending an hour in the kitchen with Belgian-born chef, Michael Stroot, is to watch a king in his castle. For Michael, preparing extraordinary food is a profession and a calling. He believes in absolutely fresh food. No dish takes more than 20 to 30 minutes to prepare and is served just as a guest sits down. He ducks out the back door for fresh herbs and does not pick the corn until the water is boiling. The stock pot on the back of the stove receives every scrap vegetable and this delicious brew is drunk as a potassium broth pick-me-up at exercise break in the morning.

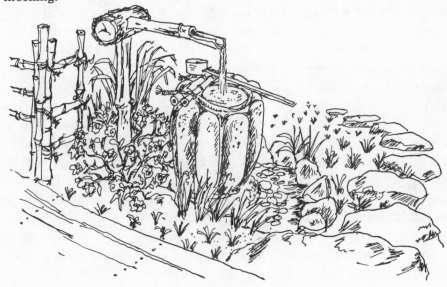

At the Golden Door each guest has a specific caloric requirement for the day, determined by Mrs. Mazzanti and staff, and adhered to by Mr. Stroot and staff. The logistics are impressive. At the end of the week, you carry home your menu, as well as recipes for preparing it. Michael Stroot holds a kitchen demonstration for recipes from the Golden Door for guests near the end of the week's stay.

The secret of the Golden Door lies in providing you with all the ingredients for a sense of your own well being. From the Japanese architecture to the carefully individualized programs, the goal is to obtain balance—a balance between exterior and interior, between activity and rest, between work and play. The result is serenity and oneness with nature—a balanced life.

It is this balance and serenity that brings guests again and again to the spa. Mrs. Mazzanti says her guests are "people who live stressfully. They have jobs which place enormous demands on their physical and emotional energy. From these tension-producing lives, they come here to get their batteries recharged, to build new reserves. . . . We get many attorneys, judges, business executives and heads of corporations." These are not people who have time to pamper themselves; they come here to unwind from the hectic world, to tune in once again to their own natural sense of balance.

The Golden Door is exclusively for women, save for certain designated weeks: Men's Weeks are conducted eight times a year, during the first two weeks of March, June, September and December. Mother-daughter Weeks and Father-son Weeks are available on a share-the-room plan June through September. Couples Weeks, one week each in March, June, September and December.

THE GOLDEN DOOR, P. O. Box 1567, Escondido, California 92025. Telephone: (714) 744-5777. Accommodations: 30 private guest rooms; private baths; telephones; television in lounge. Rates: $1250 per person, per week; special holiday rates; all meals and spa facilities included. Reservations required with $350 deposit. Inquire about mother-daughter, father-son weeks. No pets. No credit cards accepted. Open all year.
Spa facilities: steam room, sauna, Swiss hoses, indoor warm-water pool, outdoor swimming pools, tennis, dance therapy, herbal wraps, exercise program, included in lodging fees.

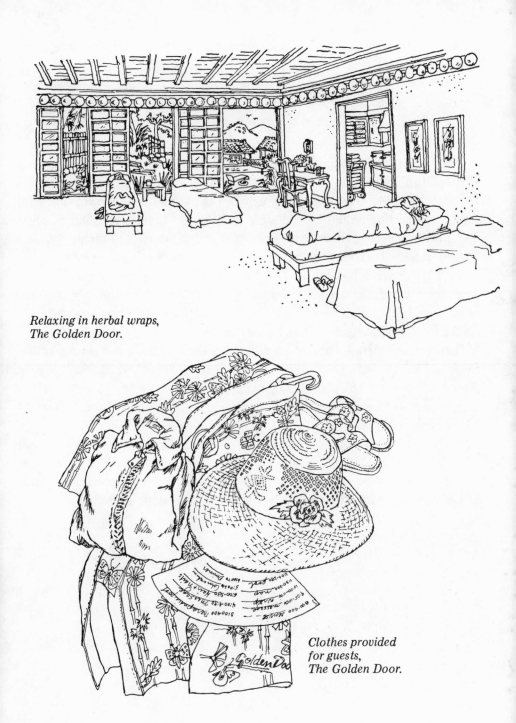

Relaxing in herbal wraps,
The Golden Door.

Clothes provided
for guests,
The Golden Door.

RANCHO LA PUERTA
Tecate, Baja California

Rancho La Puerta is the grandparent of large, health resorts in the Western United States, and continues to be judged respectfully as such after 38 years of operation. Founded in 1940 by Edmond and Deborah Szekely (now Deborah Mazzanti), the ranch has enjoyed the same administrative direction since its founding, making it possible to keep the same high quality service and health program. People return again and again to its bracing routines. Mrs. Mazzanti also founded and continues to guide the Golden Door.

Mrs. Mazzanti believes that "There is a real difference between positive good health and the absense of disease. Good health includes physical and mental health." Good health now and a blueprint for good health in the future are the objectives of Rancho La Puerta.

Rancho La Puerta is located 35 miles southeast of San Diego in the border town of Tecate, Baja California. The ranch is best reached by a scenic drive through San Diego County ranch lands (Highway 94), to the international line at Tecate. This is a quiet border crossing with no lines of traffic, and the ranch itself is only 10 minutes from the border gate.

La Puerta is situated on 150 acres of rolling countryside in a hilly terrain at 1,800 feet; the climate is mild, smogless and many classes are conducted outside. The 60 one-of-a-kind rooms range from the economical Las Casitas to Las Haciendas with living rooms, fireplaces and kitchenettes.

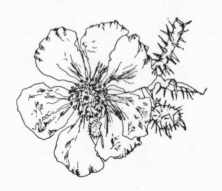

Approximately 125 guests are present each week, male and female and all ages. Children are welcome and have recreational programs of their own. The staff also numbers 125 insuring the attentive, personal service for which the ranch is famous.

The impressive facilities here include nine gyms, three swimming pools, a whirlpool-jet therapy pool, two saunas, four tennis courts, putting greens and miles of hiking trails. There are separate men's and women's centers for Swedish massage, herbal wraps, facials and scalp treatments.

A specialty of the ranch is the new fitness parcours. The first parcours, designed for specifically planned noncompetitive exercises performed in pure fresh air, was developed in Zurich, six years ago. Although there are now several hundred parcours in Europe, the idea is still new in America.

The Rancho La Puerta parcours is a six-foot-wide track about two and one-half miles in length. Placed at intervals along the track are 20 excercise stations; printed directions on the station placard prescribe the type of exercise to be performed at each stop, and whether one walks or jogs to the next station. The participant's physical condition dictates the number of times each exercise is performed. One begins with simple warm-ups, progressing to harder exercises; appropriately, the course ends with easy cool-down exercises.

The parcours is designed to improve breathing, circulation efficiency and metabolism, and generally give the benefits of cardiovascular exercise. The President's Council of Physical Fitness has recommended the parcours, and, as confirmed joggers, it is our exercise of choice at the ranch.

Daily activity schedules are tailored to your individual wishes and abilities. A typical schedule might begin with a fast morning hike at 7 o'clock, followed by stretching exercises performed under supervision for an hour, then body awareness class, Golden Door dance exercises and pool exercises. After lunch one usually schedules an individual body-conditioning program, the parcours, an hour in the pool or on the putting green, yoga, perhaps a social hour. The day ends with an evening stroll. There is no pressure on guests to keep up a regime. The atmosphere in this regard is more relaxed than most live-in fitness spas. You can enjoy as much or as little exercise as you wish, but we noticed that the great variety of activities and sports available tended to keep people occupied pleasurably all day.

The ranch diet is vegetarian, low-sodium and low-cholesterol. Although they have recently begun to serve fish one or two nights a week. Fresh natural foods grown at the ranch are served to all in the same dining room. Wonderful bread is baked daily in outdoor ovens using stone-ground wheat. Organic honey is supplied by large double hives located on the ranch, and the yogurt is delicious topped with a bit of this honey.

RANCHO LA PUERTA, Tecate, Baja California, Mexico. Telephone: (714) 478-5341 or (903) 354-1005. Accommodations: rooms and haciendas, many with fireplaces; private baths; telephones; television. Rates: $110 to $150 single, $90 to $140 per person double, for weekend; $275 to $375 single, $225 to $350 per person double, for five days, Sunday to Friday; $385 to $525 single, $315 to $490 per person double, for seven days, Sunday to Sunday; all meals and spa facilities included. Reservations required. Children welcome. No pets. Cards: AE, BA, MC, VISA. Open all year.
Spa facilities: gyms, swimming pools, whirlpool-jet therapy pool, saunas, tennis courts, Swedish massage, herbal wraps, facials, scalp treatments, parcours, included in lodging fees.

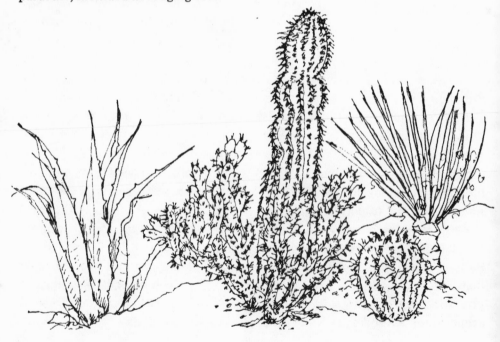

AGUA CALIENTE SPRINGS PARK
San Diego County

Agua Caliente Springs Park covers 800 acres of desert country at an elevation of 1,320 feet. Part of the San Diego County park system, the park lies in a natural amphitheater where pottery shards remain as testimony to the California Indians' long-ago use of the hot mineral-water springs. The desert flora and fauna are breathtakingly beautiful, particularly in the spring.

Although the park offers no motel comforts, there are 140 campsites from tent spaces to full trailer hook-ups, outdoor barbecue stoves, picnic tables, bathhouse, recreation building, service station, general store and post office. Visitors come from as far as 100 miles for the day to enjoy the mineral-water pools—one outdoor pool, a smaller rock-enclosed "Indian Pool" a short walk up the hill, and a glass-enclosed therapy pool with Jacuzzi. All pools are fed by the hot springs and water comes in at approximately 96 degrees. For the indoor pool, water is heated to between 98 and 102 degrees. The Indian pool is the highest in mineral content, we were told, and water temperature hovers around 86 degrees. (It feels deliciously cool on a blazing hot day.) Be warned that the Indian pool, which appears to be six to 10 feet deep, is actually much deeper; watch the children.

You know you are in the desert as you sit at one of the picnic tables in the hot sun and watch the lizards scurrying about. More charming are the antelope ground squirrels—tiny creatures with brown koala-bear noses—that burrow into the sand and pop their heads out a foot away.

There is precious little shade here and, when temperatures rise to 115 degrees during summer months, the pools close down although the park remains open. There are wonderful hiking trails with vista views of the Anza Borrego Desert.

Park systems, of course, have many rules and regulations to preserve the natural beauty of these popular recreation spots, but we shall not list them here. Their colorful brochure spells out all park rules and describes 48 parks in the San Diego system—from small historic sites to regional parks covering hundreds of acres.

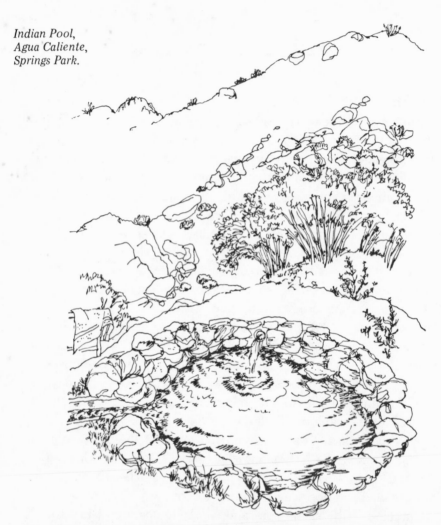

Indian Pool, Agua Caliente, Springs Park.

AGUA CALIENTE SPRINGS PARK For more information: County of San Diego Parks and Recreation Department, 1840 Weld Boulevard, El Cajon, California 92020. Telephone: (714) 475-1633. To get there: Drive east from Julian on State Highway 78 to Scissors Crossing, then south 26 miles on County S-2. Accommodations: tent space and trailer hook-ups, $4 to $5. Reservations not accepted. Youngsters under 18 must be accompanied by adults. No pets. No credit cards accepted. Park is open all year.
Spa facilities: mineral pools, no charge; 50 cents for Jacuzzi pool. Pools closed mid-July to early October.

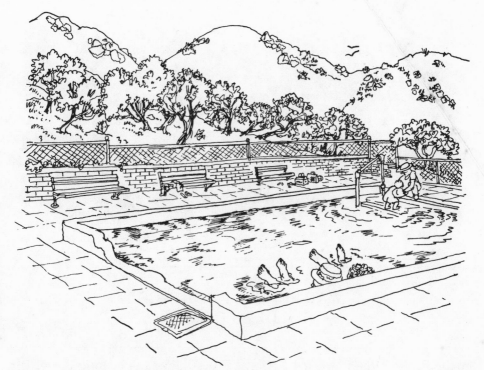

Outdoor hot mineral pool, Agua Caliente Springs Park.

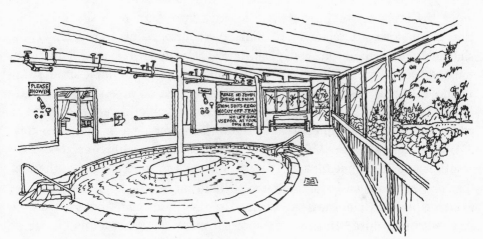

Indoor mineral pool, Agua Caliente Springs Park.

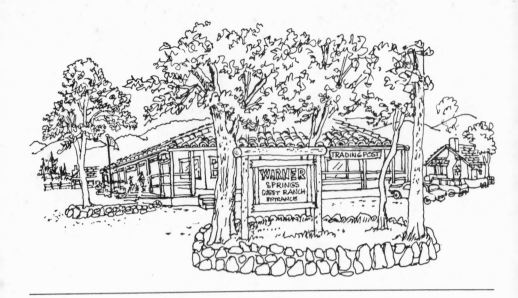

WARNER HOT SPRINGS
San Diego County

In the heart of the Cleveland National Forest along the historic Butterfield Stage Line, Warner's has retained the atmosphere of the Old West and capitalized on its Indian heritage. Charming adobe cottages with Indian names line up along dusty dirt roads. What does not reveal itself when you enter the long red-rosed, white-fenced drive into Warner's is the championship golf course, a pitch-and-putt nine-hole course, tennis courts, Ping-Pong, shuffleboard, badminton, volleyball, horseback riding trails and natural hot mineral-water springs that flow continually into two Olympic-sized swimming pools. The best of two centuries is right here. Because the spring water is continuously fed into the pools, no filters or chloride are necessary. In addition, the low-sodium content of the water makes it excellent for drinking.

Accommodations are in cottages or adobe suites with fireplaces. As a vacation and hot mineral-water resort, Warner's is superb, despite the fact that it is now owned by an absentee corporation whose appointed manager exudes a chilling aloofness in contrast to the warm and friendly old-time staff who have loved this historic spot for many years before its change of ownership. Children will find much to delight them here.

The Health Horizons Institute, under the direction of Dr. Lowell Schaeffer, operates a health program out of Warners. Literature available on request.

WARNER HOT SPRINGS, Box 10, San Diego County, California 92086. Located north of Santa Ysabel on Highway 79. Telephone: (714) 782-3555. Accommodations: cottages, one-, two- and three-bedroom suites; private baths; no telephones; no television. Rates: cottages $24 to $36, suites $40 to $62. Dining room with full bar service. Deposit required with reservation. Children welcome. $7.50 per night charge for pets. Cards: AE, BA, MC. Open all year.
Spa facilities: hot mineral-water swimming pools, no charge for overnight guests.

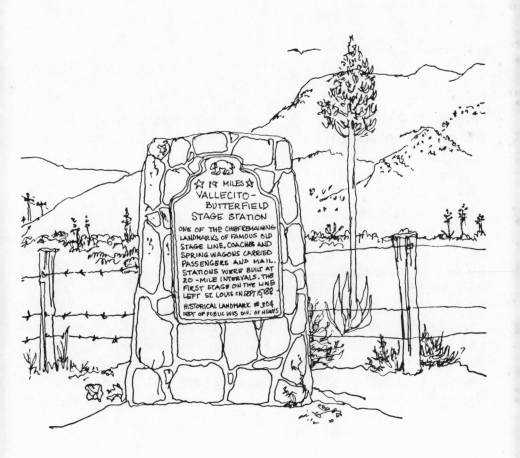

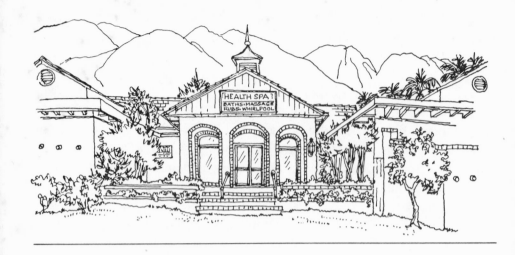

MASSACRE CANYON INN
Gilman Hot Springs, Riverside County

Massacre Canyon Inn and the old pink stucco bathhouse across the highway recall many eras of colorful California history. MCI, as it is called, is advertised today as a complete recreational facility with a 27-hole golf course, tennis courts, coffee shop, evening dining and entertainment, swimming pool and a self-contained health spa—now far removed in time and spirit from the event that gave the inn its name.

Massacre Canyon in the foothills of the San Jacinto mountains was the site of a tragedy that exterminated an entire tribe of Indians. The Ivah Indians had lived peacefully on the site of the present spa, gathering their chia (a type of sage, the seeds of which were eaten) that grew abundantly on the heights above the canyon. When one of California's periodic droughts wiped out the chia supply of the neighboring war-like Temeculas, they massacred the entire Ivah tribe in order to obtain their chia.

Apparently, the commercialization of the hot springs began in 1881 when the spa was named Mineral Relief Springs and advertised as equal to the famous German spas in Baden-Baden. In 1913, a family named Gilman discovered the healing waters and purchased the land. At that time, there was a small hotel, a few cottages, an old wooden bathhouse and mud holes for bathing. The Gilmans rebuilt the bathhouse and, according to old-time spa staffers, rebuilding has been going on ever since.

The present bathhouse, across the road from the inn, was constructed in 1955. A clipping on the bulletin board sets the mood of the spa: "The magic of the mineral water ... if you suffer from arthritis or rheumatism ... will improve your circulation, tone your muscles and relax tension."

The spa facility sectioned into men's and women's quarters, is rustic, spartan and spacious. A small lobby is at the center of the building with tub, sauna and massage facilities contained in two enormous rooms to each side. Six individual, contoured black-and-white tiled tubs line one wall, each with its portable Jacuzzi planted outside like a canister vacuum cleaner; shower curtains can be drawn across the tub for privacy.

The spa still offers salt rubs and blanket wraps in curtained cubicles that fill the center of the floor space. The austere surroundings do not detract from the luxurious feeling of a rub-down. The sauna is a good-sized room maintained at approximately 160 degrees. The rock stove is fenced in for safety and a small pan of water and ladle are close by so that you can lower

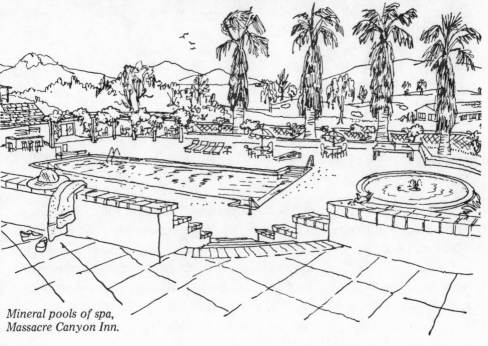

Mineral pools of spa,
Massacre Canyon Inn.

the temperature whenever you choose. The mud baths, sadly, are no longer used, but do take a look at the mud-bath room, one of the few in southern California. At the front of the spa building facing "MCI," both women's and men's sections have an outdoor sundeck enclosed by high concrete siding for nude sunbathing.

A large gymnasium is in a separate structure behind the spa and has been used for many years by famous boxers who come to MCI for their spring training. Manager Mike Penrod will be glad to list off the boxing stars who have trained here, and you might, as we did, run into heavyweight champs like Ken Norton.

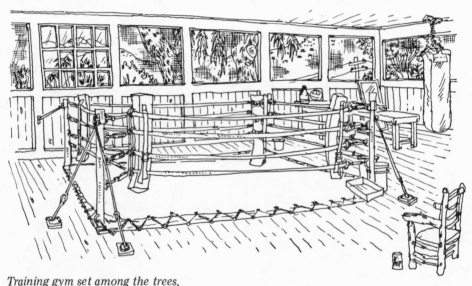

Training gym set among the trees,
Massacre Canyon Inn.

MCI does not incorporate a "spa program" in their rates. A variety of room accommodations are available and all spa services are "à la carte." MCI offers vastly different vacation experiences, depending upon your accommo-dations: The Inn offers unpretentious motel rooms and down-home friendli-ness for those who want to golf, dine, dance, and swim; on the spa side of the highway there are rustic adobes for those who want to spend their time nurturing, indulging and invigorating a tired body. Or one may enjoy a smorgasbord by playing both sides of the street!

MASSACRE CANYON INN, Gilman Hot Springs, California 92340. Telephone: (714) 654-7301. Accommodations: "rancho" and "villa" rooms and suites on spa side; "lodge" rooms and suites on inn side; private baths; single and double beds; telephones; television. Rates: $18 to $36. Coffee shop, dining room, full bar service. Children welcome. No pets. Cards: AE, BA, MC, VISA. Open all year.
Spa facilities: mineral tubs, $5; whirlpool, $5; salt rub, $4; steam room and sundeck, $3; massage, $10.

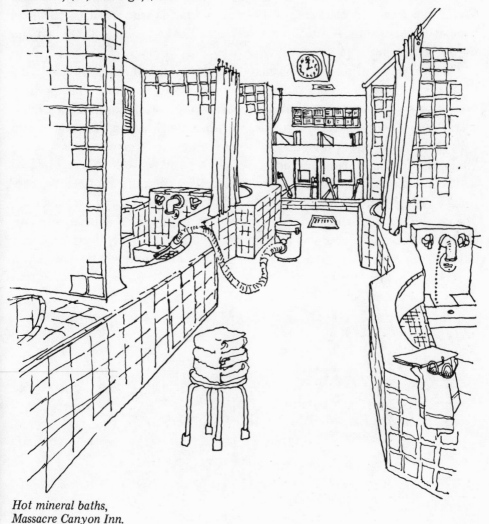

Hot mineral baths,
Massacre Canyon Inn.

HIGHLAND SPRINGS RESORT
Beaumont, Riverside County

When purchased in 1884 by Dr. Isaac Smith, this resort was called the Highland Home Hotel. Now encompassing some 1,600 acres surrounded by the beautiful snow-peaked San Jacinto mountains, it is owned by Howard Rosen and expertly managed by Bill and Nora Zilz who describe Highland Springs Resort as the "Catskills of the West." The elevation is 3,000 feet and the air is marvelous.

There is an unmistakable elegance to the grounds and the hotel itself, and a vastness that would take more than a day to explore, and that, perhaps best done on horseback. Activities include a large swimming pool, a smaller therapy pool with jet sprays, tennis, golf, horseback riding, horseshoes and volleyball. Elaborate programs from hay rides to weiner roasts can be arranged, on request, for children.

The bathhouse—closed when we visited—is a magnificent facility; contoured tile tubs and walls sparkle with reds, turquoises and yellows, and each private tub room is distinctively different in its art deco adornment. This enormous room also contains a "heat box"—literally a box, lined with heat lamps, from which the head protrudes through an opening in the top, like a

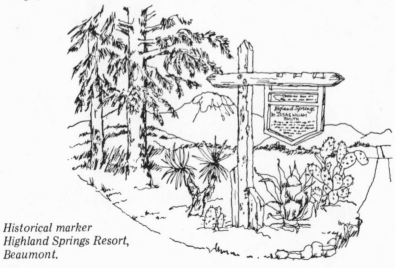

Historical marker
Highland Springs Resort,
Beaumont.

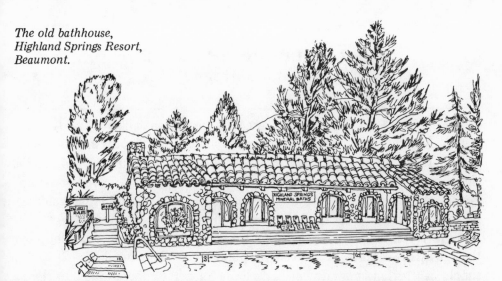

The old bathhouse,
Highland Springs Resort,
Beaumont.

character from Alice in Wonderland. We then found a room with a "sitz bath" chair, a beautiful redwood sauna and massage rooms. Touring the old bathhouse was like discovering a treasure in the attic. When Highland Springs re-opens its full spa facilities, it will be the envy of the area.

Highland Springs operates on the American Plan, serving two meals a day in their spacious dining rooms next to their cocktail lounge. The food is beautifully prepared and their desserts are tantalizing. There is a wide range of variability in the accommodations offered, from individual cottages to lodge rooms.

While the resort itself is a self-contained hideaway, Palm Springs is only 20 minutes away and Hemet is easily accessible in the other direction. Oak Glen "apple country" is close by, and is a must stop for apple pie lovers.

HIGHLAND SPRINGS RESORT, Beaumont, California 92223. Telephone: (714) 845-1151 or (213) 271-5505. Accommodations: cottages and lodge rooms; private baths; twin and double beds; no telephones; television. Rates: $32 to $114 cottages, $69 to $87 rooms, two meals included. Restaurant with full bar. Children welcome. No pets. No credit cards accepted. Open all· year.
Spa facilities: large outdoor swimming pool, small whirlpool; no charge for overnight guests. Bathhouse, not open at present, has sauna, tub, sitz bath and heat cabinet.

PALM SPRINGS SPA HOTEL
Palm Springs

In the mid-1800s, Palm Springs was an Indian village called SeKhe (boiling water). A bathhouse for stagecoach travelers was operated on the site of the present Palm Springs Spa, built in 1960. The hotel was built in 1963 and a third story—the limit imposed in this desert area—was added in 1965. Mineral water from the spa's own well feeds into two 50,000-gallon storage tanks and is reheated for use in the spa facility.

As lovely as the Palm Springs Spa Hotel is, we were pleased to find that the spa itself is open to the general public on a daily-use basis. One may simply call for an appointment or walk in for a hot mineral-water swirlpool bath, rock steam bath, vapor inhalation therapy, use of the gymnasium, facial and/or complete body massage—all at reasonable cost. The outdoor mineral-water "therapy" pools located in a pavilion between the spa and the hotel may also be enjoyed for a daily fee. Hotel guests have all spa privileges once daily, gratis, with the exception of massage and facial, and may use the outdoor therapy pools in addition to the very large swimming pool.

Palm Springs Spa.

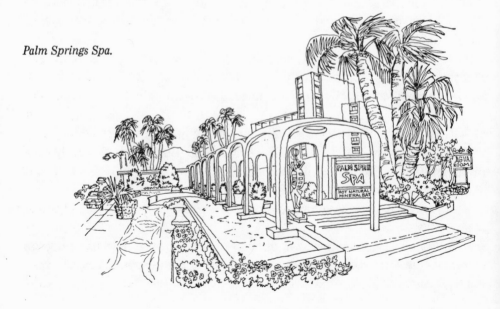

Bathhouse at Palm Springs Spa.

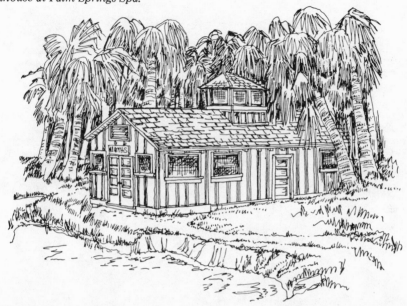

The spa has been expertly run by Marguerite Byerly for many years. There are men's and women's sections offering duplicate services; the gymnasium is co-ed and is accessible from both sections. The spa provides guests with private dressing rooms and a bright red cotton jersey sweat suit for working out in the gym.

You are free to do your own exercises using all the standard gym equipment provided, *or* you may consult with Arnie Dahlen who has presided over the gym for some time and knows his stuff. His background and interests are in physical medicine; if you suffer from chronic back pain, do tell him, for he has a fine set of orthopedic exercises that are not only easy to accomplish but require no equipment. He knows the dangers of pushing yourself beyond your physical capacity and has a gentle and non-competitive approach to exercise regimes.

After changing out of your gym suit, you will don paper scuffs and a large wrap-around towel and an attendant will usher you about. Although you may go through the spa's activities in whatever order suits you, the staff recommends that you proceed from the gym to the "inhalation" room, warm but not blistering hot, where wonderful vapors assail your nostrils.

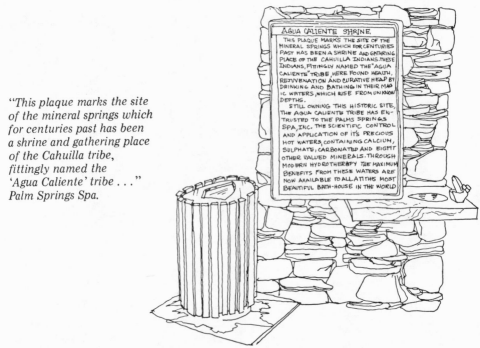

"This plaque marks the site of the mineral springs which for centuries past has been a shrine and gathering place of the Cahuilla tribe, fittingly named the 'Agua Caliente' tribe . . ."
Palm Springs Spa.

Next spend a short sojourn in the spacious rock steam room (maintained at 160 degrees) and then sink into a contoured tile tub, located in private rooms with beaded curtains, for your whirlpool bath. (If you prefer a very hot tub—106 degrees—call ahead and ask that the water not be drawn until the moment you are ready. Those opting for a somewhat cooler tub, can have it drawn ahead of time.

After your bath, you can either shower or go on to the cooling room where an attendant will wrap you in a soft cotton sheet, place cool-dipped gauze pads over your eyes, and leave you on a cot to rest and relax for whatever length of time you specify. We recommend that you *not* pass up the cooling room—the relaxation you will feel here, after your workout and tub soak, is worth all the tranquilizers you can buy. Guests generally schedule their facial and/or massage at the end of their day's activities.

If your main interest is to soak in hot mineral water and relax in the sun, the outside mineral-water pools are quite lovely and you can move back and forth from hot to hotter, resting on a poolside chaise between dips. Should you want to avoid the hot sun, try the large glass-enclosed pool to the rear of the outside pools.

The service desk at the hotel supplies information on tours, the desert museum, Living Desert reserve, botanical gardens, date ranches, horseback riding, hiking, biking and, of course, the Palm Springs Aerial Tramway that takes you up 8,500 feet over the desert to the top of Mt. San Jacinto.

PALM SPRINGS SPA HOTEL, P.O. Box 1787, Palm Springs, California 92262. Telephone: (714) 325-1461 or (800) 472-4371. Accommodations: one-room executive suites with wet bars; one- and two-bedroom luxury suites with bar and kitchen; private baths; twin beds; telephones; color television. Rates: $58 to $165, $30 to $90 in summer. Dining room with full bar service. Deposit required with reservation. Children welcome. No pets. Cards: AE, BA, DC, MC, VISA. Open all year.
Spa facilities: outdoor mineral pools, whirlpool mineral baths and bath-house facilities, no charge to overnight guests. Day use: mineral baths with rock steam, vapor inhalation, cooling room and gymnasium, $6; massage with mineral bath and gym, $15; massage only, $10 for one-half hour, $15 for 45 minutes; outdoor mineral pools, $5. Inside bathhouse open 9 am to 5 pm; bathhouse closed June 12 to September 21.

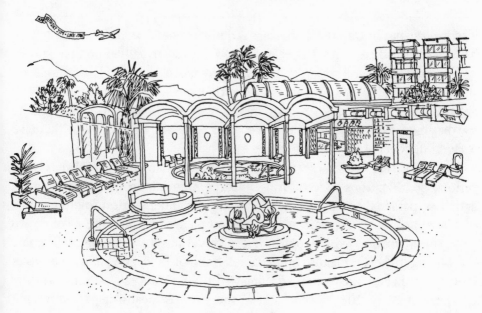

Hot mineral pools in the courtyard, Palm Springs Spa.

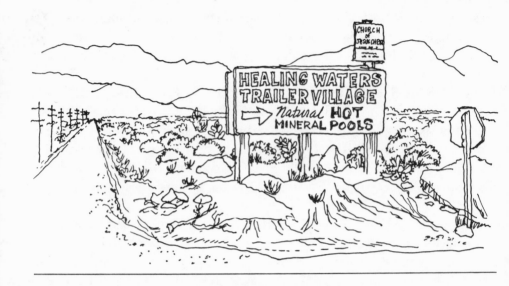

DESERT HOT SPRINGS
Riverside County

The health spas in Desert Hot Springs require a general word of introduction. This beautiful desert city has been blessed with a virtually unlimited supply of natural hot mineral water, and most of the motels have their own wells on the property. The "spa" facilities are neither those of a La Costa, where all activities are individually programmed, nor of a Gilman Hot Springs where the bathhouse is a structure that dates back to early settlers and the *agua caliente* discovered by the Indians.

You will find in Desert Hot Springs more than 100 motel-spas with various combinations of creature comforts, entertainment, gung-ho health activities, personal pampering, healing mysteries and historical folklore.

These motel-spas are built on a common plan of an inner-pool courtyard or pavilion surrounded by rooms. *Every* motel has a swimming pool where the temperature is cooled to approximately 85 or 90 degrees and each has at least one "therapeutic" pool, equipped with whirlpool jets, at temperatures of approximately 104 degrees. Those that feature health-spa facilities are, with few exceptions, a complex of spa *services* located inside the courtyard that you use on a do-it-yourself basis. Many do not have a masseur or masseuse on the premises, but you almost always can make an appointment at the motel desk for a masseur to come to you—either to the massage room available or to your hotel room and sometimes even to the outside pool area, should you want your massage out in the sunshine.

A number of motels in the area display a "Spa-Tel" sign. The Spa-Tel Association was formed essentially to maintain quality standards in Desert Hot Springs' motel-spa facilities. The two rules for membership are that you have a well on your premises and that the temperature of the water comes out of the ground at 100 degrees or more. The higher the temperature, the more impurities surface and, thus, the higher the mineral content. We also learned that it costs $5,000 to sink a well. We began asking the various places we visited whether thay had their own well, but stopped when the answer was an invariable "yes." Without delving into the local politics of the situation, we can only say that *not* belonging to the Spa-Tel Association does not mean that there is no well on the premises. Obviously, not all motel-spas saw advantages to Spa-Tel membership.

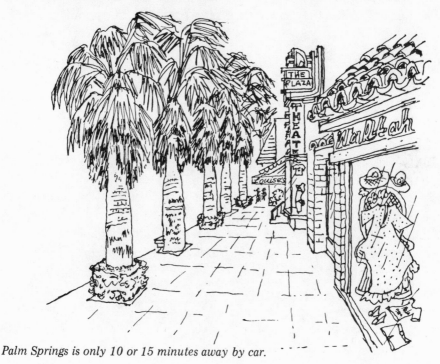

Palm Springs is only 10 or 15 minutes away by car.

Because of the uniformity of motel-spa design throughout Desert Hot Springs, we have selected to feature those that are distinctive—either in the way their spa package is put together or in the kinds of accommodations they offer. In doing so, we have passed over many excellent motels—no matter how lovely they may be—if they do not offer a bit more than the standard two pools and a motel room.

Most saunas in this area are dry heat—do not be deceived by the attractive rocks and sprinkle water on as you would in San Francisco's Finnish sauna.

Owners and managers of motel-spas in Desert Hot Springs, as elsewhere in the southland, constantly shift. They also constantly spruce up and often expand their facilities, so be a bit wary of their colored brochures; some will give you a true picture, but others will not. To print new brochures with each change would not be feasible.

The summer months (June to October) are off season in the desert area, for temperatures soar to 110 and 115 degrees. This is the time when most motel-spa owners fix up their facilities, refurbish and install new indoor-outdoor carpeting that is so rapidly eaten away by the mineral water. Of course, it is also the time when they lower their rates for those hardy souls who take

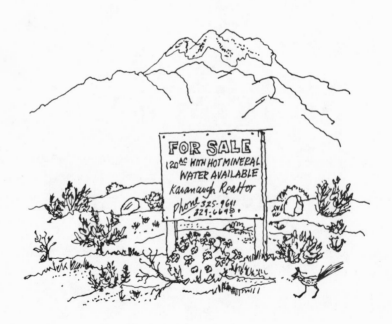

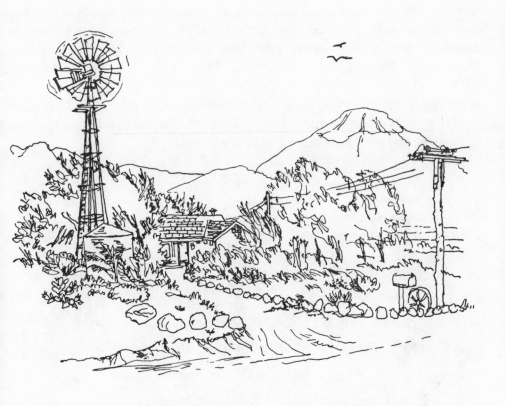

well to the heat. The afternoon winds come up in the desert around four o'clock and bring welcome relief from the blistering heat. Temperatures remain very warm into the evening and night, however, and sitting out at 11 o'clock up to your neck in 90- or 104-degree water is exquisitely pleasant and soothing. (Mineral water is unbelievably soft and makes your skin feel like baby velvet to the touch.) If you are not accustomed to desert heat, be sure to moderate your activities for a few days, to stay inside during mid-day sun, and to sip water frequently throughout the day. You are most likely going to be drinking mineral water as well as soaking in it, and you should not gulp it down in huge quantity until your body has had a chance to get used to it.

Palm Springs is only 10 or 15 minutes away by car and offers an entirely different atmosphere. Here the majesty of mountains takes precedence over the vast stretches of desert sand, and the city life sparkles in contrast to the soporific pleasures of Desert Hot Springs. But do watch out for sand storms as you cross the desert strip into Palm Springs; they can be fierce and frightening, although usually short-lived. There is limousine service to most Desert Hot Springs spa-motels from the Palm Springs Airport.

Desert Hot Springs Chamber of Commerce operates a tourist information center described as "unequalled anywhere." We suggest you talk with them if you plan to spend some time in this desert region.

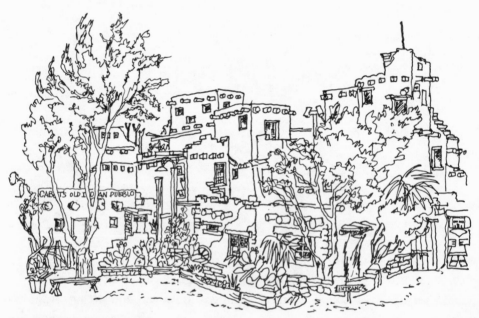

Cabot's Old Indian Pueblo,
now a museum,
near Desert Hot Springs.

DESERT INN
Desert Hot Springs

Desert Inn Hotel and Spa does not reveal its splendor from the outside. But when you open the glass door from the main lobby and gaze out at the pool pavilion you will know that you have come upon the super spa of Desert Hot Springs. There are *eight* pools in varying temperatures and as you move about from blissfully cool to womb-warm to hot to hottest you feel like Goldilocks in the House of Three Bears looking for the one that's "just right."

All pools and the various spa services in the pavilion (sauna, massage, showers, beauty shop) are open to the public on a day-use, pay-for-services basis. Although the public may use the pools until 10:30 in the evening, hotel guests can wander out from their poolside room at midnight and find a group of friendly soakers smoothing away the last wrinkle of tension before bedtime.

The people using the spa facility are wonderfully variegated: a young father instructing his daughter in Spanish as she traverses the ledge in one of the cooler pools while mother stretches out on a chaise nearby; a bevy of bronzed young people planning their evening, signing the heavy plaster cast on the leg of one of their friends; youngsters diving in and out of the Olympic-size swimming pool or playing in the specially designed children's pool; a young bearded man, eyes closed to the sky, meditatively alone in another circular pool; an older gent's shock of white hair bobbing out of one of the hotter pools.

For the number of people using pool facilities during the day, the noise level is surprisingly low. The pool area is also kept scrupulously clean—despite the availability of food service at poolside on weekends. Small palm trees break up the expanse of concrete and large penguins sit patiently about, pretending they are trash cans.

The sauna room is good size with long redwood benches and an electric coil oven topped with rocks. As with most spas, massage appointments must be made at the desk and massage is not included (as are all other services) in

133

the hotel guest privileges. Desert Inn also offers a guest card to a private 18-hole golf course, tennis courts and horseback riding in the area.

Part of the Desert Inn complex is a restaurant, the International Trophy Room, that features nightly entertainment; there is also a bright, gay, blue-green-white coffee shop where "George," one of the roadrunners native to the desert, comes to the door for his morning treat from one of the waitresses.

If you want a free, convivial atmosphere for your soaking and body relaxation, a wide choice of water temperatures, and all creature comforts, this is the place.

The two-story hotel has 50 rooms, facing the pool pavilion; all have king- or queen-size beds and color television. While it is convenient to stay in a downstairs room where your glass sliding doors open right to the pools, if you prefer a bit more privacy from this public area, you may want to reserve an upstairs room.

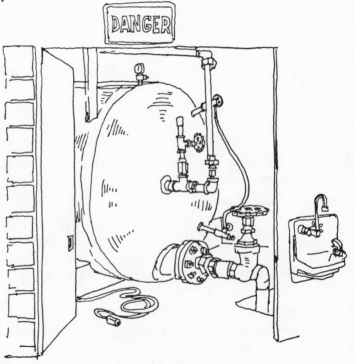

The holding tanks for hot mineral water, Desert Inn Hotel and Spa.

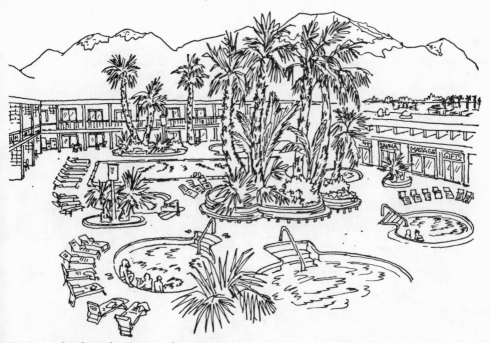

Eight pools of varying temperatures,
Desert Inn Hotel and Spa.

The manager of Desert Inn is a young, perky woman who makes you feel like an instant friend and seems to know many guests by name, stopping to talk with them by the pool. The ownership of Desert Inn Hotel and Spa is changing, but we believe that the manager and her warm and friendly staff will remain, sending out the "good vibes" that make such a difference in how a place feels.

DESERT INN HOTEL AND SPA, 10805 Palm Drive, Desert Hot Springs, California 92240. Telephone: (714) 329-6495. Accommodations: hotel rooms and suites; private baths; twin, double, twin double, queen- and king-size beds; telephones; color television. Rates: $35 to $65; lower weekly and summer rates. Coffee shop, dining room, full bar service. Deposit required with reservation. Children welcome. No pets. Cards: AE, BA, DC, MC, VISA. Open all year.
Spa facilities: eight pools, sauna, $5 for day use, no charge to hotel guests·
massage, $10 for one-half hour by appointmen

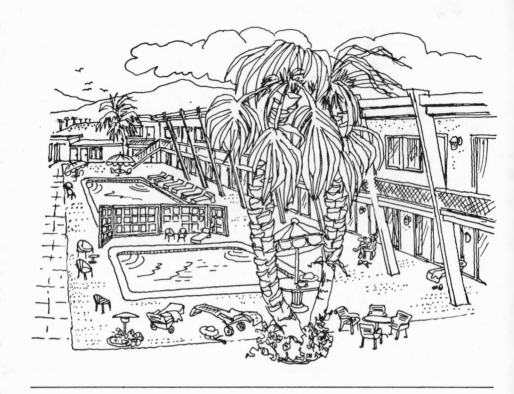

LINDA VISTA LODGE
Desert Hot Springs

A connoisseur of Desert Hot Springs may wonder why we are including Linda Vista Lodge which appears to be very much on a par with many other good motels we have passed over. Essentially, we felt that you should know about one more place that has a very inviting resort facility for families. In addition to a 50-foot swimming pool and interior hot therapy pools, Linda Vista has a miniature golf course (lighted in the evening), a fine recreation room with Ping-Pong and billiards, and an outdoor shuffleboard.

There is also a shaded coffee area near the pool where you can get out of the sun and relax a bit. The motel is very compact and parents should feel quite comfortable here enjoying the hot mineral waters, the lovely rock steam room and sauna while the children occupy themselves in their own activities. As at the Desert Inn Hotel and Spa, we saw a three-generation family—child, father and grandfather—all having a wonderful time together in the pool. Another special facet of Linda Vista is that they permit pets on a leash.

The motel-spa has 42 units, 30 with kitchens, in some cases connecting two units so that two families can share the kitchen and still have the privacy of their rooms. Some rooms have sunken tubs and all have color television.

LINDA VISTA LODGE, 67200 Hacienda Drive, Desert Hot Springs, California 92240. Telephone: (714) 329-9000. Accommodations: motel rooms, some connecting; private baths; no telephones; color television; some rooms with kitchens. Rates: $21 to $28; lower weekly, monthly and summer rates. No meal service; coffee area and soft-drink machines. Deposit required with reservation. Children welcome. Pets permitted on leash. Cards: BA, MC, VISA. Open all year.
Spa facilities: swimming pool, Jacuzzi/therapy pool, steam room, no charge to hotel guests. Masseur available by appointment.

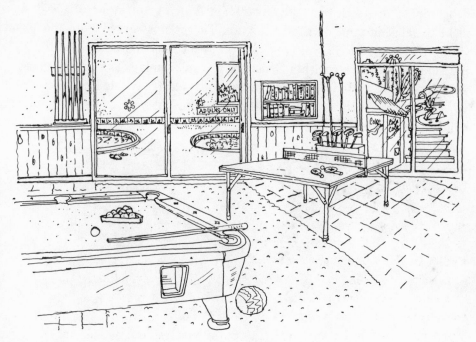

Linda Vista Lodge,
Desert Hot Springs.

PONCE DE LEON HOTEL
Desert Hot Springs

The "high-rise" in Desert Hot Springs, the Ponce de Leon is a three-story structure with a penthouse suite. Under new management, this Best Western hotel wraps its 107 units around an inner courtyard containing three mineral-water pools—one for swimming and the others (one outside and one enclosed) for hot water soaking. The therapy pools with whirlpool jet action are equipped with in-pool chairs. As at the Desert Inn Hotel and Spa, health spa services are all contained within the pool pavilion—a redwood sauna, massage rooms and small beauty shop, but here they are open to hotel guests only. The hotel also has its own coffee shop.

Ponce de Leon is the only hotel in the area that offers private therapy pools with some of its rooms; this is its distinctive feature. Imagine the delight of slipping through a glass sliding door at any hour of the day or night to relax in your own private pool. The pool is lighted from above and within and you can control its jet action by a timing meter. Behind the pool is a small outside area with a chaise for private sunning. The television set in your room is mounted on a swivel pole so it is clearly visible from the pool if you don't want to miss your favorite program, but your body is crying for relief from a strenuous desert hike.

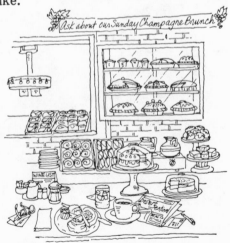

Coffee shop, Ponce de Leon Hotel in Desert Hot Springs.

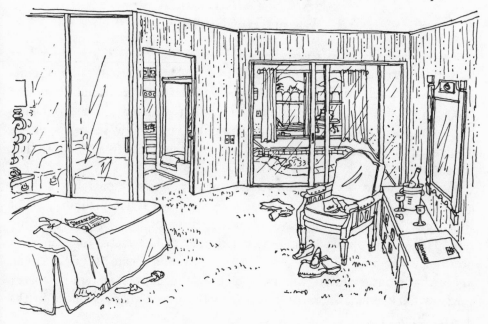

Room with private hydro-jet mineral pool and garden, Ponce de Leon Health Spa.

This is also the only hotel in Desert Hot Springs with a penthouse suite—an ultra-modern, spacious unit with three-plus bedrooms and the added touch of a bidet in your bathroom.

PONCE DE LEON HOTEL AND HEALTH SPA, 11000 Palm Drive, Desert Hot Springs, California 92240. Telephone: (714) 329-6484 or (800) 528-1234. Accommodations: hotel rooms, one- and two-bedroom suites with full kitchens, private-pool rooms, penthouse; private baths; twin, queen-, king-size and water beds; telephones; television. Rates: rooms $28 to $36; suites $30 to $70; private pool rooms $50 to $60; lower rates in summer, fall and for groups. Coffee shop. Deposit required with reservations. Children welcome. Small pets permitted. Cards: AE, BA, CB, DC, MC, VISA. Open all year.
Spa facilities: swimming pools, jet therapy pools, sauna open to hotel guests only at no charge; massage by appointment, $10 for one-half hour, $15 for one hour.

139

SAM'S FAMILY SPA
Desert Hot Springs

If you are traveling with young children and don't want the restraints that are inevitable in any motel/hotel, you may want to think about the sprawling family-style campground and resort situated on the outskirts of Desert Hot Springs. Sam's has three hot mineral-water wells on its 40-acre property and boasts continuous pumping of "fresh flo-thru hot mineral water."

In addition to its swimming and soaking pools, Sam's has a large game room, recreation hall, general store and self-service laundry, all of which can be used by the day, by overnighters, or on a weekly/monthly rate. This AAA-approved campground is one place where you can soak up the water and sunshine, enjoy the vast and beautiful desert, and know that your children will have plenty to occupy their young energy —even a duck pond where they can feed the quack-quacks. Ducks in the desert? Yep!

Sam's provides above-average camping and trailer-park facilities, but do not expect luxury in the motel rooms and mobile-home units.

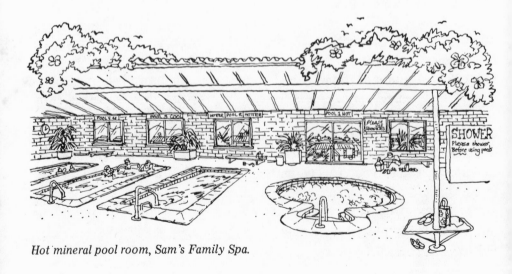

Hot mineral pool room, Sam's Family Spa.

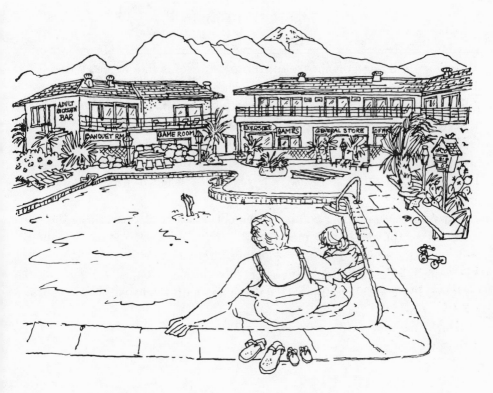

SAM'S FAMILY SPA AND HOT WATER RESORT, 70-85 Dillon Road, Desert Hot Springs, California 92240. Telephone: (714) 329-6457. Accommodations: facilities for travel and tent trailers, campers, motor homes and mobile homes; motel rooms and mobile home units; no telephones; some with kitchens. Rates: $10 to $13 per day, $125 to $155 per month for recreational vehicle hook-ups; $25 to $45 per day for motel rooms and mobile-home units; weekly and monthly rates available. No meal service; snack bar and general store. Reservations not accepted on camper spaces; reservation with deposit required for motel rooms and mobile-home units. Children welcome. No pets. No credit cards accepted. Open all year.
Spa facilities: swimming pool, four hot pools, exercise room, $4 for day use; no charge for overnight guests.

SPA TOWNHOUSE
Desert Hot Springs

We include the Spa Townhouse for those who would like to spend their time in a little more privacy and quiet than the larger places provide and enjoy a Desert Hot Springs vacation at a very modest price. As you approach the Townhouse you are likely to find owner-manager Melanie Koosli watering her lawn by the outdoor pool in plain view from the street. Melanie moved here with her husband and son in 1977 and they are trying to bring the Townhouse back to its beauty of years past when it was frequented by movie stars.

Grassy areas are not a common sight in Desert Hot Springs, so the lawn surrounding the pools is something of a novelty, as is the open L-shaped design of this motel. Behind the main swimming pool is a therapeutic hot water pool enclosed by fencing but open to the sky. Bougainvillea drapes the motel building which contains 10 units, some with kitchens. Black and white

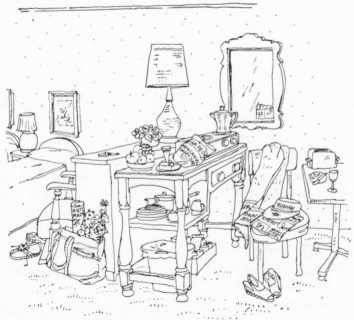

Making yourself at home, Spa Townhouse

The Spa Townhouse, Desert Hot Springs.

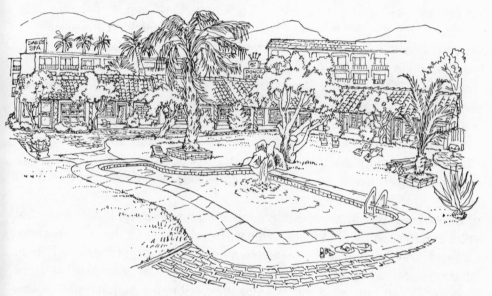

cable television in each room, a soft-drink machine and a barbecue area complete this little gem. Restaurants and night life are a hop, skip and a jump away, as are the public spa facilities of the Desert Inn Hotel and Spa. By the way, Melanie teaches crafts and you should ask to see her fabulous bread sculpture.

SPA TOWNHOUSE, 6540 East Sixth Street, Desert Hot Springs, California 92240. Telephone: (714) 329-6014. Accommodations: three-room apartments and efficiency units with refrigerator and hot plate; private baths; no telephones; television. Rates: $18 to $22, plus $3 to $4 for extra-person occupancy. No meal service; barbecue area and soft-drink machine. Deposit required with reservations. Children welcome. Small pets permitted. No credit cards accepted. Open all year.
Spa facilities: swimming pool and therapeutic pool open to hotel guests only at no charge.

THE WHITE HOUSE
Desert Hot Springs

An imposing mosque-like structure, The White House is one of the few spas in Desert Hot Springs that has been under one ownership for the past 25 years. It is small (eight units) and, as owner Bill Green describes it, "the toughest spa in town."

Green tours each of his guests through the spa when they arrive. As he puts it, he can "hand-pick" his guests and beam his business to those who want pure rest and relaxation. To that end, he is strict about his rules and regulations: no children, no pets, no hoop-la—the front entrance closes at 10:30. He candidly describes his running commentary for the tour as a canned speech—"please do not ask any questions until I have completed the tour."

Beyond the small motel lobby, the outdoor courtyard shelters a hot mineral-water soak and a "cool" plunge. In the corner of the pool area is an enclosed structure housing a good-sized indoor pool equipped with switch-on jet sprays located at nine different body levels in the water so that every limb and joint can receive their massaging, vibrating action. Also in this enclosure is a very attractive sauna that guests reserve by paying 25 cents at the front desk. Madness? No. Bill Green insists on knowing when someone is in the sauna, since many people still do not realize that there is a strict limit to the length of time one should remain in its intensive heat.

Green is also strict about the general "no lotions" rule that is posted in all mineral-water pool facilities. Lotions leave a contaminating film on the water and while you might assume that people would be considerate of each other in this respect, many seem oblivious to the "no lotions" signs, or, justifiably, they are more concerned that they do not burn. It is possible, however, to pop into the shower just before entering the pool and to apply lotion again once you have finished your hot soak. The White House was the only spa in this area that seemed to enforce the regulation. (A number of spas sell a Shaklee lotion that contains no oils and is apparently acceptable in most places.)

All of the rooms at the White House open onto the pool pavilion and, though not "posh," have a spartan sweetness to them reminiscent of a New England boarding house. In fact, guests are asked to make up their own beds until a linen change is provided. There are four fully equipped kitchens. No eating is permitted in the rooms; however, a shaded, plant-lined solarium just off the main courtyard is equipped with a long table and chairs, an ice machine and a coffee maker—an inviting place to share a lunch or snack with other guests.

Green concludes his tour with other "house rules": You always take a towel with you to the pool area (towels are "endlessly provided"); you always dry yourself and your suit before entering your room; and you help yourself to the giant-sized bottle of Bactine standing staunchly on one of the poolside tables. With the explanation of Bactine's presence as the only "after-soak lotion" allowed, the tour is at an end.

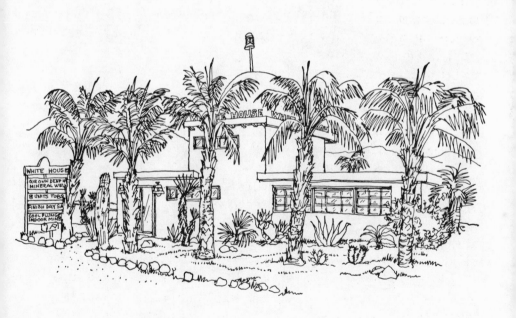

The White House, Desert Hot Springs.

Tough? Not for everyone? Right. But if you are over 21, want no nonsense, noise or frills with your mineral-water vacation in this lovely desert town, you will like it here and you will get along with Bill Green just fine.

THE WHITE HOUSE, 11285 Mesquite Avenue, Desert Hot Springs, California 92240. Telephone: (714) 329-7125. Motel rooms; private baths; twin and double beds; some kitchens; no telephones; no television. Rates: $18 to $19, kitchens $2 extra, weekly rates. No meal service. Deposit required with reservation. Children not permitted. No pets. No credit cards accepted. Open all year.
Spa facilities: hot and cool plunge, indoor hydro-jet mineral pool, sauna, no charge for motel guests.

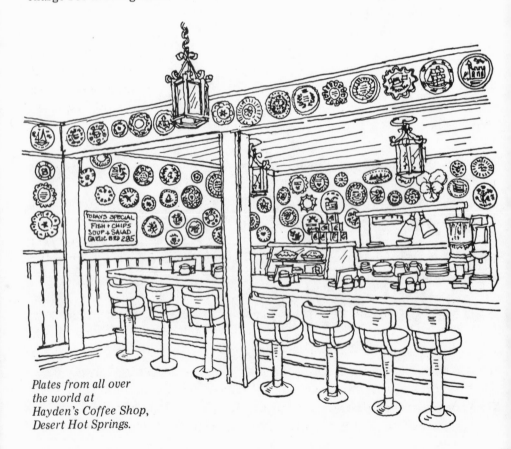

*Plates from all over
the world at
Hayden's Coffee Shop,
Desert Hot Springs.*

TWO BUNCH PALMS
Desert Hot Springs

Every guidebook has to have its "big find"—the place you happen upon and want to keep all to yourself. Two Bunch Palms is ours. It can hardly be kept a secret, however, for when we discovered it they were completely restoring, renovating and expanding their facilities in order to be ready for the opening of the season. Two Bunch certainly will not attract those who want all of the comforts of a hotel at their fingertips—rooms have no telephones and there is no restaurant. That may be why it has been a favorite hideaway for writers and is frequented by television performers and crews who need a get-away-from-it-all place plus the amenities offered body, mind and soul.

Two Bunch Palms does not show from the road, and the road itself is not in the main motel section of town. You turn off Two Bunch Palms Drive onto a dirt trail; although a sign is posted, the first sure indication that you've arrived is a view of two bunches of palm trees in the distance. The story goes that government surveyors of the desert area in the 1850s spotted the dramatic palm trees in two distinct clusters with an inviting passageway between and marked it on their map as "Two Bunch Palms." Then, as the tale goes, they left a note under a rock saying "Too damned hot—going to mountains."

The area has been well planted in the last four or five years. Now, unlike most of Desert Hot Springs, Two Bunch offers considerable shade from the hot sun. Beautiful tamarisk trees rustle fiercely in the afternoon wind, rising to a pitch that mimics the ebb and flow of the ocean and soothes the troubled mind.

Two Bunch Palms offers historical, visual and atmospheric contrasts to the other spas in Desert Hot Springs and, indeed, to those in the state. Its known history starts in the 1930s when Thomas Lipp built the still-standing "Rock House" for his family dwelling. In 1945, the structure that now houses the main lounge, snack bar, game room and bathhouse, was a gambling casino. At that time, such movie greats as Alice Faye, Errol Flynn and Jack Dempsey would come here to gamble and to take the waters and salt rubs.

It was even rumored that Al Capone had spent time in the Rock House, although Peter Warner, the spa's energetic manager of the last three years, admits that the story is unlikely since the chronology of the spa and that of Capone's imprisonment simply don't fit. He obviously enjoys the story, however, and will tell you that the two suites in the Rock House have been named the "Al Capone" suite and the "Bugsy Siegel" suite. The splendid collectors-item safe built into the wall in the downstairs bathhouse is testimony enough that notorious underworld figures frequented Two Bunch in its casino days. Gambling was outlawed in the desert in 1948.

Visually, your first glimpse of the pool area will make you wonder whether you are still in Desert Hot Springs. At the bottom of a few rock steps is a long stretch of grotto-like pool whose water is incredibly blue. The pool area is graced on one side by lovely flora and fauna and on the other by a rocky expanse with picnic tables, a recessed barbecue section and massive outdoor fireplace. A few motel units (that more resemble small cottages than the usual motel) face the pool-picnic area. The general rockiness of the area and the lush foliage, jasmine, oleander and tamarisk trees, set the inviting tone of Two Bunch. The quiet is broken only by the constant gurgling of the hot mineral water as it flows into the pools from their well one-quarter mile up the hill.

A cement "bench" immersed along the circumference of the pool allows you to sit and dangle your feet or to safely lower yourself down into the soft, pale blue water. Follow the gurgling noise over to the spigot nestled in the rocks and feel the blistering heat of the water as it comes into the pool.

What appears to be one pool is, in fact, two. As you move along its length, you will wade around a large foliated center planter to a smaller pool almost hidden in the rear. The water here is 106 degrees and the inside walls are equipped with jet sprays that you operate from a timing meter just above the pool. According to Manager Warner, their water comes in at 165 degrees and flows freely into the pools, continuing through a by-pass that runs in front of the Rock House and thence out to the desert.

The hideaway atmosphere of days past has so far been retained by the large land development firm that now owns Two Bunch. At the time we visited, Peter Warner showed us around and pointed out all of the renovations that were to be completed within the next few months. The upstairs living room in the old casino building was brimming with velvet and mahogany pieces of unknown vintage, waiting, along with 400 stored antiques,

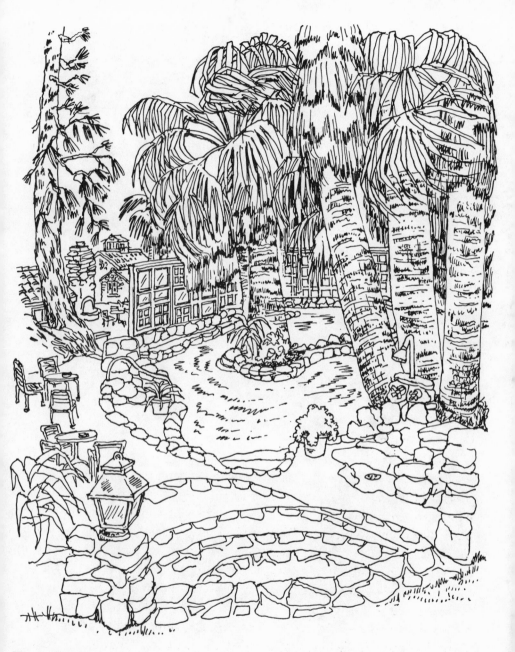

The pools at Two Bunch Palms,
Desert Hot Springs.

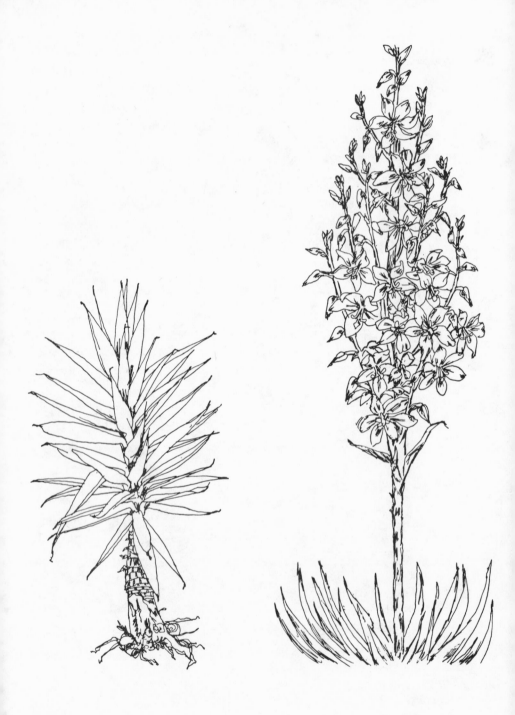

for the decorator to transform this salon into its past elegance. A pool table stood incongruously alone, waiting for its future home. A sun porch off the living room overlooks the condominium units and the 230 acres of desert land that make up Two Bunch Palms' property. A small room to the side is to become a snack bar.

The spa facilities are in a large basement room behind a small counter that once must have served as a bar. There are six massage rooms, private tub rooms with brightly colored tiles painted with art-deco motifs, and a lovely tiled sauna.

Beyond the casino-bathhouse, opposite the pool area, is a huge expanse of land that is to encompass two tennis courts (with tournament level lighting), a large exercise pool for "aquabics," a volleyball court, and what the Marines call "circuit training" or weight-lifting. Obviously, there is no way that this idyllic spot is going to remain a secret.

Accommodations are equally distinctive—from single motel rooms furnished with antique four-poster beds and highboys, to modern shag-rugged condominiums with kitchens, to the magnificent Rock House containing two two-bedroom suites and an upstairs deck with small wet bar and outside bathroom/shower.

It is simply not possible to describe adequately this desert jewel. Did we tell you about the rabbit who sits outside the door? The hummingbirds? The meditation area between the two bunches of palms?

TWO BUNCH PALMS, 67-220 Two Bunch Palms Drive, Desert Hot Springs, California 92240. Telephone: (714) 329-8791. Accommodations: motel rooms, one- and two-bedroom condominiums with kitchens; two-bedroom suites with living room and kitchen; private baths; no telephones; no television. Rates: $25 to $35 without kitchen, $35 to $75 with kitchen, $80 to $100 suites; continental breakfast included. No other meal service, snack bar. Deposit required with reservation. Children under 16 not permitted. No pets. No credit cards accepted. Open all year.
Spa facilities: All bathhouse and recreational facilities—use of pools, salt rubs, exercise courts, volleyball, aquabics—included for motel guests. Massage $10 for one-half hour by appointment.

WALDORF HEALTH RESORT
Desert Hot Springs

In a separate category from the other motel-spas in this area is the Waldorf, which offers an extensive therapeutic program on a week-long basis. Hanni Dorf, who has owned the resort for the past 18 years, has elaborate plans for remodeling their spacious facility. The main building is unimposing from the outside, but the rear building is a striking sight; the upper floor is completely glassed in and looks out on an expanse of desert. When we visited, this structure was being totally refurbished to house a large gymnasium, recreation room, massage rooms and an impressive red-tableclothed dining area with a magnificent view.

Included in the week's program are desert walks, daily sun baths, mineral-water therapy in three hot mineral-water pools, exercise and yoga classes, facials and massage in addition to three lecture/discussions per week on the art of preparing natural foods. Weight reduction is one of the Waldorf's specialties and all food prepared in their "Golden Dorf" kitchen is organically grown and invitingly served. Fasting is also possible at the Waldorf; all fasting and dietary programs are worked out in consultation with Dr. Jonathan Spector, a chiropractor and naturopathic physician.

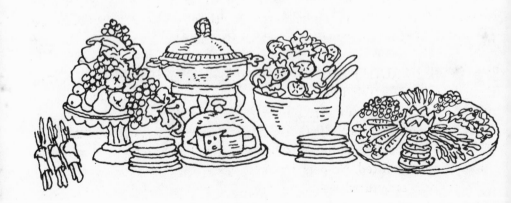

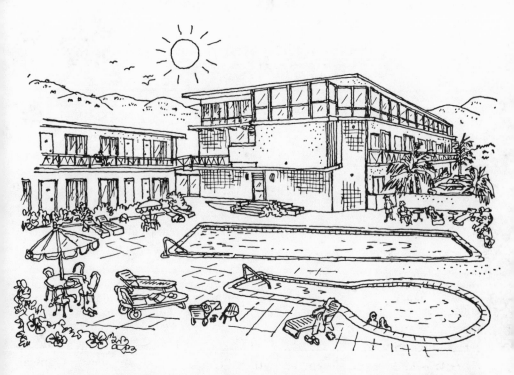

The atmosphere here is warm and friendly, and we would tend to believe that the Waldorf is, indeed, an "oasis of health, friendship, and pleasures," as their one-page "fact sheet" proudly proclaims. It concludes that "For what you would pay for a bleak hotel room you can afford the opportunity to get well, stay well, with T*L*C: tender, loving care."

Their prices bear out that statement. For all of the services included in the weekly rate of $150 to $200, we found it to be reasonable. But it does presume that you want a structured health program and that you are comfortable with a naturopathic approach to health.

WALDORF HEALTH RESORT, 1190 Mesquite Avenue, Desert Hot Springs, California 92240. Telephone: (714) 329-6491. Accommodations: motel rooms; private baths; some refrigerators, some kitchens; some telephones; television. Weekly rates: $150 per person, double occupancy; $200 per person, single occupancy; meals included. Deposit required with reservation Children not permitted. No pets. Cards: BA, MC, VISA. Open all year.
Spa facilities: structured week-long program only; included in weekly rates.

INDEX

Agua Caliente Springs Park, 113-115
Alameda County, 66-75
Albany, 66-69
Albany Sauna, 66-69
Alt Karlsbad, 13
Ambassador Tennis and Health Club, 90-91
American Family Sauna and Hot Tub, 70-72
Aquabics, spas with, 83, 95, 99, 104, 110, 147
Ashram, The, 88-89

Baja California, 110-112
Basic bag, 7, 9
Beaumont, 122-123
Berkeley, 73-75
Berkeley Sauna, 73-75
Big Sur, 79-81
Blanket/herbal wraps, spas with, 19, 22, 32, 36, 99, 104, 110, 118

Calistoga, 15-41
Calistoga Spa, 19-21
Campbell Hot Springs, 50-52
Camping facilities, spas with, 47-50, 94, 113, 140
Carlsbad, 13, 99-103
Colusa County, 42-46
Corona, 92-94

Dance exercises, spas with, 83, 95, 99, 104, 110
Desert Hot Springs, 128-153
Desert Inn Hotel and Spa, 133-135
Diet programs, spas with, 83, 88, 95, 99, 104, 152
Disco dance, 100-101
Dr. Wilkinson's Hot Springs, 22-25

Esalen Hot Springs, 79-81
Esalen massage, 80
Escondido, 104-109
Exercise programs, spas with, 83, 88, 95, 99, 104, 110, 124, 147, 152

Fallbrook, 95-98
Family Sauna Shops, 53-57
Finnish sauna, information on, 10, 53-54

Gilman Hot Springs, 118-121
Glen Ivy Hot Springs, 92-94
Glen Ivy Recreational Vehicle Park, 94
Golden Door, The, 104-109
Golden Haven Spa, 26-28
Grand Central Sauna and Hot Tub, 58-60
Gymnasiums, spas with, 61, 88, 90, 99, 110, 118, 124, 152

Herbal wraps, spas with, see blanket wraps
Highland Springs Resort, 122-123
History of California spas, 10, 12, 15, 16, 37, 76, 147-148

Japanese baths and massage, 10, 61-64

Kabuki Hot Spring, 61-64

La Costa Spa, 99-103
Linda Vista Lodge, 136-137
Los Angeles, 88-91

Massacre Canyon Inn, 118-121
Massage, information on, 28, 46, 80
Mendocino County, 47-48
Mineral-spring water, information on, 16, 26, 76
Monterey County, 76-81
Mountain Home Ranch, 29-31
Mud baths, information on, 16, 20-21, 22-23, 34
Mud baths, spas with, 19, 22, 32, 36, 92

Nance's Hot Springs, 32-35
Napa Valley, 15-41

Oakland, 70-72
Oaks at Ojai, 83-87

154

Ojai, 83-87
Orr Hot Springs, 47-48

Pacheteau's Original Calistoga Hot
    Springs, 36-39
Pala Mesa Resort, 95-98
Palm Springs area, 122-153
Palm Springs Spa Hotel, 124-127
Parcours, 111
Physical therapy, spas with, 22, 40
Ponce de Leon Hotel and Health Spa,
    138-139

Rancho La Costa, 99-103
Rancho La Puerta, 110-112
Recreational vehicle facilities, spas with,
    94, 113, 140
Reflexology foot massage, information
    on, 28
Richmond, 70-72
Riverside County, 92-94, 118-153
Roman Spa, 40-41

Salt rubs, spas with, 118, 147
Sam's Family Spa and Hot Water Resort,
    140
San Diego County, 95-109, 113-117
San Francisco, 53-65

Saunas, information on, 53-54, 68, 75
Shiatsu massage, 10, 62
Sierra County, 50-52
Sierraville, 50-52
Soboba Hot Springs, 13
Spa programs, 83, 95, 99, 104, 110, 152
Spa Townhouse, 142-143
Swedish saunas, 75
Swiss showers, spas with, 99, 104

Tassajara Hot Springs, 76-78
Tecate, 110-112
Tipping, 6
Trailer facilities, see recreational vehicle
    facilities
Two Bunch Palms, 147-151

Ukiah, 47-48

Waldorf Health Resort, 152-153
Warner Hot Springs, 116-117
Water temperature, 9
White House, The, 144-146
Wilbur Hot Springs, 42-46
Wilbur Springs, 42-46

Yoga classes, spas with, 42, 83, 88, 90,
    99, 104, 152

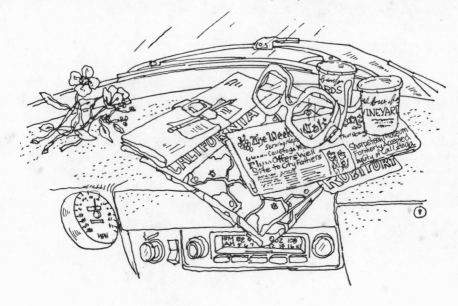

BIOGRAPHICAL NOTES

Mutually shared interests in health, the outdoors and travel brought together the collaborators on this book. All are residents of Berkeley and spend much of their time exploring California's countryside—and "taking the waters."

PATRICIA COOPER is an educator, research biologist and author of several other books, as well as numerous articles for women's magazines and scientific publications. At the University of California she has taught courses in human development and women's health. Her other books are *The Quilters* (Doubleday, 1976) and *Woman's Body: A Health and Medical Guide,* to be published in 1979 by Meredith Press.

LAUREL COOK is an editor and free-lance author. For 10 years she was scientific editor at the University of California, and later was assistant to the director of a new medical program, sponsored by the university and its medical center in San Francisco. She is presently working as an editor and manuscript consultant on several health and medical books.

FRAN ATTAWAY is an artist, designer and craftsperson. A former New Yorker, she has specialized in the design of record albums for major recording companies; has worked in Japan, as a design and advertising consultant; in Bali, as a marketing advisor to native craftsmen; and for 11 years lived in Barbados, West Indies, where she devoted most of her time to crafts in all media. She produces a weekly crafts column *Make It* for the *San Francisco Chronicle.*